FAQs on

RATIONAL ANTIBIOTIC THERAPY

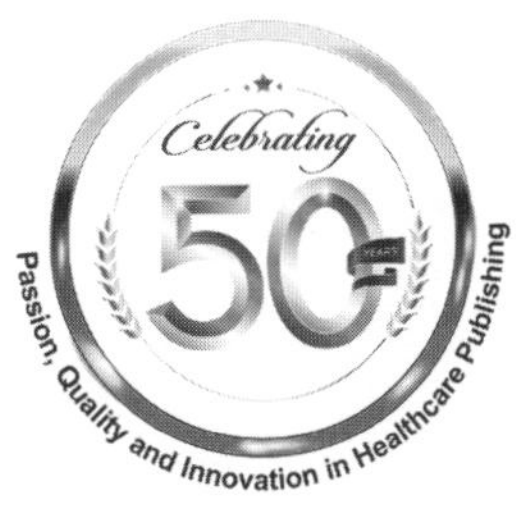

FAQs on
RATIONAL ANTIBIOTIC THERAPY

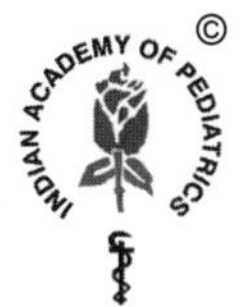

Editors-in-Chief

Abhay K Shah
MD (Ped) (Gold Medalist)
DPed (UNI FIRST) FIAP
Senior Consultant Pediatrician
Children Hospital
Ahmedabad, Gujarat, India
Member ACVIP
Advisory Committee on Vaccines and Immunization Practices
Indian Academy of Pediatrics (IAP)(2018–19)
Chairman, Infectious Diseases Chapter of IAP 2015

Digant D Shastri
MD (Ped) FIAP PGDHHM
CEO and Senior Pediatrician
Killol Children Hospital
Surat, Gujarat, India
President
Indian Academy of Pediatrics

Editors

Jaydeep Choudhury
DNB (Ped) MNAMS FIAP
Associate Professor
Department of Pediatrics
Institute of Child Health
Kolkata, West Bengal, India
Vice President (East Zone) CIAP, 2019

Parang N Mehta
MD (Pediatrics)
Consultant Pediatrician
Mehta Hospital
Surat, Gujarat, India
Editor, Bulletin of Infectious Diseases, 2004–2009
Member, IAP Committee on Immunisation, 2007–2008

Forewords

Digant D Shastri
Santosh T Soans

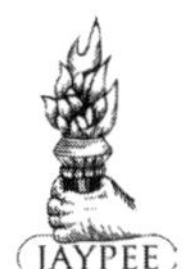

JAYPEE BROTHERS MEDICAL PUBLISHERS
The Health Sciences Publisher
New Delhi | London | Panama

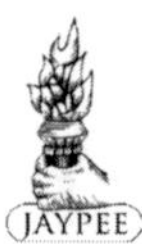

Jaypee Brothers Medical Publishers (P) Ltd.

Headquarters
Jaypee Brothers Medical Publishers (P) Ltd.
4838/24, Ansari Road, Daryaganj
New Delhi 110 002, India
Phone: +91-11-43574357
Fax: +91-11-43574314
Email: jaypee@jaypeebrothers.com

Overseas Offices

JP Medical Ltd.
83, Victoria Street, London
SW1H 0HW (UK)
Phone: +44 20 3170 8910
Fax: +44 (0)20 3008 6180
E-mail: info@jpmedpub.com

Jaypee-Highlights Medical Publishers Inc.
City of Knowledge, Bld. 235, 2nd Floor, Clayton
Panama City, Panama
Phone: +1 507-301-0496
Fax: +1 507-301-0499
E-mail: cservice@jphmedical.com

Jaypee Brothers Medical Publishers (P) Ltd.
Bhotahity, Kathmandu, Nepal
Phone: +977-9741283608
E-mail: kathmandu@jaypeebrothers.com

Website: www.jaypeebrothers.com
Website: www.jaypeedigital.com

Inquiries for bulk sales may be solicited at: jaypee@jaypeebrothers.com

FAQs on Rational Antibiotic Therapy

First Edition: **2019**

ISBN: 978-93-5270-968-7

Printed at: Rajkamal Electric Press, Kundli, Haryana.

Dedication

This book is dedicated to children of our great nation, all teachers and seniors who guided us, and all members of our beloved academy.

CONTRIBUTORS

Abhay K Shah
MD (Ped) (Gold Medalist) D Ped (UNI FIRST) FIAP
Senior Consultant Pediatrician
Children Hospital
Ahmedabad, Gujarat, India
Member, Advisory Committee on Vaccines and Immunization Practices (ACVIP)
Indian Academy of Pediatrics (IAP) (2018-19)
Chairman, Infectious Diseases Chapter of (IAP) 2015

Amarjeet Chitkara
MD DNB FIAP
Director and Head
Department of Pediatrics
Max Superspeciality Hospital
New Delhi, India

Aniruddha Ghosh
MD
Senior Resident
Department of Pediatrics
Institute of Child Health
Kolkata, West Bengal, India

Ashok Rai
MD PhD FIAP FIAMS FNNF FACI
Consultant Pediatrician
Surya Super Speciality Hospital
Varanasi
Kilkari Institute of Child Health Private Limited
Varanasi
Director, Indian Institute of Cerebral Palsy and Handicapped Children
Varanasi
Honorable IMA Professor of Pediatrics and Faculty, Heritage Institute of Medical Sciences
Varanasi, Uttar Pradesh, India

Baldev S Prajapati
MD (D Ped) (Gold Medalist) FIAP MNAMS FICMCH
Head and Professor
Department of Pediatrics
GCS Medical College, Hospital and Research Centre
Ahmedabad
Aakanksha Children Hospital and Postgraduate Institute
Ahmedabad, Gujarat, India

Bharat Mehra
MD
Fellow (Intensive Care)
Sir Ganga Ram Hospital
New Delhi, India

Bhaskar Shenoy
MBBS MD (Ped) Diploma in PID FAN
Head
Department of Pediatrics
Chief
Division of Pediatric Infectious Diseases
Manipal Hospital
Bengaluru, Karnataka
Adjunct Professor (Pediatrics)
Manipal University
Bengaluru, Karnataka, India

Chetan Shah
MD
Chief Pediatrician and Neonatologist
Anand Children Hospital
Surat, Gujarat, India

Dhanya Dharmapalan
MD PG Dip in PID (Oxford)
Consultant (Pediatric Infectious Diseases)
Apollo Hospitals
Navi Mumbai, Maharashtra, India

Digant D Shastri
MD (Ped) FIAP PGDHHM
CEO and Senior Pediatrician
Killol Children Hospital
Surat Gujarat, India
President
Indian Academy of Pediatrics

Janani Sankar
MBBS DNB PhD MAMS
Senior Consultant Pediatrician
Kanchi Kamakoti CHILDS Trust Hospital
Chennai, Tamil Nadu, India

Jaydeep Choudhury
DNB (Ped) MNAMS FIAP
Associate Professor
Department of Pediatrics
Institute of Child Health
Kolkata, West Bengal, India
Vice President (East Zone) CIAP, 2019

Jeeson C Unni
MD DCH
Editor-in-Chief
IAP Drug Formulary
Chairperson, IAP Neurodevelopment Chapter
Senior Associate Consultant in Pediatrics
Aster Medcity
Kochi, Kerala, India

Ketan H Shah
MD (Ped)
Private Practitioner
Ketan Children Hospital
Visiting Doctor
Surat Municipal Corporation
Saachi Hospital, Mahavir Hospital
Surat, Gujarat, India

Kheya Ghosh Uttam
MD DNB (Ped)
Assistant Professor and NICU-In-Charge
Department of Pediatrics
Institute of Child Health
Kolkata, West Bengal, India

Narayanappa D
MD (Ped) FIAP
Professor
Department of Pediatrics
JSS Medical College
JSS Academy of Higher Education and Research
Mysuru, Karnataka, India
Chairman, IAP-ID Chapter, 2019

Nupur Ganguly
DCH DNB (Ped) FIAP
Associate Professor
Department of Pediatrics
Institute of Child Health
Kolkata, West Bengal, India

Parang N Mehta
MD (Ped)
Consultant Pediatrician
Mehta Hospital
Surat, Gujarat, India
Editor, Bulletin of Infectious Diseases, 2004–2009
Member, IAP Committee on Immunization, 2007–2008

Pratima Shah
MD Dped
Consultant Pediatrician
Ankur Institute of Child Health
Ahmedabad
Former Professor and HOD
Medical College
Vadodara, Gujarat, India

Rajal B Prajapati
MD (Ped) DPed
Professor (Pediatrics)
VS General Hospital and AMC MET Medical College
Ahmedabad, Gujarat, India

Raju C Shah
MD DPed FIAP FRCPCH (UK)
Medical Director
Ankur Institute of Child Health Ahmedabad
Former Professor and Head
Department of Pediatrics
GCS Medical College
Ahmedabad, Gujarat, India

Ritabrata Kundu
MD
Professor
Department of Pediatrics
Institute of Child Health
Kolkata, West Bengal, India

Ritesh Shah
MD (Ped)
Fellowship (Pediatric Neurology)
SAACHI Children Hospital
Surat, Gujarat, India

Sanjay K Ghorpade
MD (Ped)
Director and Professor
Department of Pediatrics
Post Graduate Institute of Pediatrics and
Niramay Hospital and Research Center
Satara, Maharashtra, India

Santanu Bhakta
MD DCH FIAP
Senior Consultant Pediatrician
Kolkata, West Bengal, India

Shyam Kukreja
MBBS DCH MD (Ped)
Director and Head
Department of Pediatrics
Max Super Specialty Hospital
New Delhi, India

Suchi Acharya
MBBS MD (Ped)
Senior Resident
Institute of Child Health
Kolkata, West Bengal, India

Upendra Kinjawadekar
MD DCH
Consultant Pediatrician and
Neonatologist
Kamalesh Mother and Child Hospital
Navi Mumbai, Maharashtra, India

Vijay Yewale
MD (Ped) DCH FIAP
Head
Institute of Child Health
Apollo Hospitals, Navi Mumbai
Director
Dr Yewale Multispecialty Hospital for
Children
Navi Mumbai, Maharashtra, India

Vipin Goyal
MD DCH
Consultant Pediatrician and
Neonatologist
Kamalesh Mother and Child Hospital
Navi Mumbai, Maharashtra, India

FOREWORD

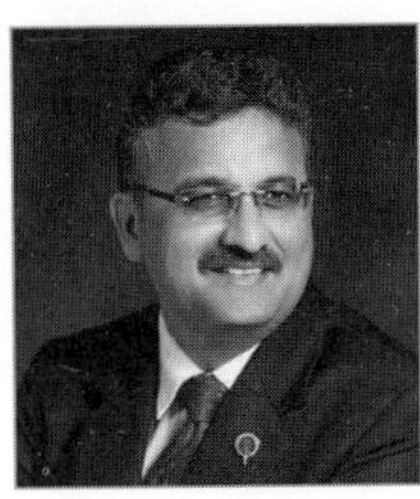

It is a proud privilege for me to write the foreword for the first edition of Indian Academy of Pediatrics (IAP) publication of *FAQs on Rational Antibiotic Therapy*.

Antibiotics are one of the most significant therapeutic reserves of the medical history. Proper selection of antibiotics is a multifaceted process that requires careful clinical judgment but unfortunately, selection and the use of antibiotics is made lightly without regarding to the therapeutic features of the drug and to the infecting microorganisms. The wide use of antibiotics has been associated with increasing antimicrobial resistance, both in the community and hospital settings. Patient care is threatened by treatment failure arising from infection of organisms leading to morbidity and potential mortality. The treatment of these infections is hampered by the lack of efficacious antibiotics, especially for multi-resistant gram-negative organisms like *Acinetobacter* and *Pseudomonas aeruginosa*. Furthermore, widespread abuse and overuse of antibiotics result in potential drug toxicities leading to increased complications as well as increased healthcare costs.

Looking to the magnitude of problem of irrational antibiotic therapy by doctor, it has been planned by IAP to publish book on *FAQs on Rational Antibiotic Therapy*.

In the current publication, all important aspects of rational antibiotic therapy for various pediatric infections are being addressed very diligently in FAQ format. The book covers details of various antimicrobial agents, rational management of various infections and also antimicrobial formulary.

My sincere compliments and congratulations to all the authors who as a part of their since efforts to disseminate the knowledge, have contributed chapters for this prestigious publication. I congratulate the entire editorial board lead by Dr Abhay K Shah, Dr Parang N Mehta, Dr Jaydeep Choudhury for their untiring efforts to bring out this book.

I am sure that this book will be popular amongst the postgraduate students, teaching faculties as well as practicing pediatricians. I wish this landmark publication great success and wish it will contribute in minimizing menace of misuse/abuse of antimicrobials.

Digant D Shastri
President
Indian Academy of Pediatrics, 2019

FOREWORD

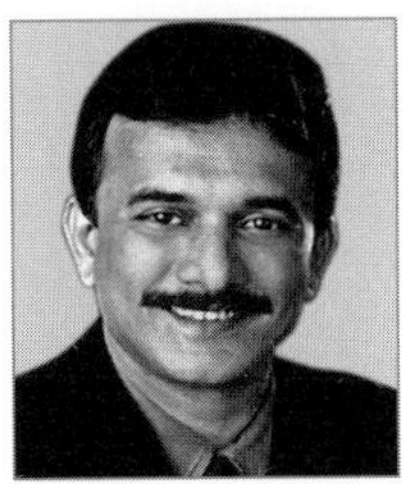

I am delighted to know that *FAQs on Rational Antibiotic Therapy* have been compiled under the editorial stewardship of Dr Abhay K Shah, eminent pediatrician and Dr Digant D Shastri, President, IAP, 2019 who are very active in IAP Infectious Disease chapter and has contributed in many ways. They are ably supported in this endeavor by editors Dr Jaydeep Choudhury and Dr Parang N Mehta who are both active members of Infectious Disease chapter. I am happy to say that they have brought out this comprehensive book in record time which I am sure will be loved by academicians. This is a remarkable and commendable achievement. I wish to congratulate all colleagues involved in this monumental effort.

Frequently asked questions (FAQs) are listed questions and answers, all supposed to be commonly asked in some context and pertaining to a particular topic. The format is commonly used on e-mail mailing lists and other online forums, where certain common questions tend to recur. Busy practitioners are confronted with many questions which need to be answered immediately and may be difficult to find in textbooks. This FAQs book will definitely help them to find the answers immediately.

Rational antibiotic use requires accurate diagnosis and appropriate antibiotic use. Antibiotics have radically improved the prognosis of infectious diseases. Infections that were almost invariably fatal are now almost always curable if treatment is started early. Antibiotics are among our most valuable resources, but their use is threatened by the emergence of resistant strains of bacteria. Physicians need to use antibiotics wisely and responsibly. This means that when deciding which antibiotic to use, we need to consider the likelihood that an antibiotic will induce resistance, as well as traditional evidence-based comparisons of efficacy.

I wish the readers an enlightening academic experience. I am sure this book is going to be a darling of IAPians and hope to see next edition as soon as possible.

Santosh T Soans
President
Indian Academy of Pediatrics, 2018

PREFACE

FAQs is the abbreviation of frequently asked questions; literally it means a list of questions and answers relating to a particular subject, especially one giving basic information for the readers. The purpose of this book is to highlight important and relevant questions and answers to the readers as the busy pediatric practitioners often find it difficult to get the answer to the questions in the midst of bulky texts. These FAQs have been collected from discussions in various forums. Many important issues pertaining to infectious diseases have been illustrated through concise and well-written chapters in the form of FAQs which cover basic knowledge about the disease, its diagnosis, and management. Besides being evidence based, the book is written by experts in the field of pediatric infectious diseases from all over the country. The contents have been drafted keeping up with the advancements in the pediatric subspecialty. Care has been taken to include infections that are common in our country and also emerging and re-emerging infections.

It is a privilege that this book is being published during Pedicon 2019 in Mumbai. It is a great forum to reach many pediatricians. The ultimate success of the book depends on the acceptance and usefulness of this book to the readers. We believe this book will serve as a desktop handbook and ready reference for commonly encountered situations in pediatric infectious diseases.

Editorial Board

ACKNOWLEDGMENTS

The members of editorial board are highly thankful to all the contributors and reviewers for their academic contributions. Our special thanks to office bearers, executive board members of Indian Academy of Pediatrics for their permission to bring out this book.

We are thankful to Shri Jitendar P Vij (Group Chairman), Mr Ankit Vij (Managing Director), Ms Chetna Malhotra Vohra (Associate Director—Content Strategy), Dr Savleen Kaur (Development Editor) and the team of M/s Jaypee Brothers Medical Publishers (P) Ltd, New Delhi, India, for giving a go-ahead at the very beginning and helping us in every way possible to bring out this book.

CONTENTS

SECTION 1
General Considerations

SECTION 2
Common Infections in Office Practice

SECTION 3
Healthcare-associated Infections and Special Situations

SECTION 4
Superbugs

SECTION 5
Salvaging the Antibiotics

SECTION 6
Annexures

SECTION 1

General Considerations

- Basics of Rational Antibiotic Practice
- Failure of Antibiotic Therapy
- General Principles in Antibiotic Therapy
- Adverse Effects of Antibiotics and Its Management
- Chemoprophylaxis

CHAPTER 1

Basics of Rational Antibiotic Practice

Raju C Shah, Pratima Shah

Q1. "Inappropriate use of antibiotics" is an often heard term. What does this mean?

All forms of antibiotic misuse and abuse are termed as "inappropriate use of antibiotics". When antibiotics are taken for too short a time, at too low a dose, at inadequate potency, or for the wrong disease one can call it inappropriate use.

Q2. Why do we need judicial antibiotic practices?

Worldwide infectious diseases are still a serious problem. Development of antibiotic resistance in many bacteria has now compounded it. Pipeline of development of newer antimicrobial agents to combat these multi-resistant organisms has dried up in last decade.

Evidence shows that prescriptions of broad-spectrum antibiotic have increased and are prescribed frequently when either no therapy is necessary or when narrower-spectrum alternatives are appropriate. Respiratory conditions most of which are viral for which more than 10 million antibiotic prescriptions per year are generated which are unlikely to provide any benefit.

Q3. Is it a serious threat to mankind?

A patient admitted with bacterial infection to hospital is expected to be cured by first-line antibiotics. If this patient is infected with multi-resistant organism, could get a serious infectious disease, which fails to respond to commonly and regularly used antibiotics and his/her stay in the hospital could be very long.

Such treatment failure can lead to severe complications, as the infection spreads to all or few other systems of the body which will need intensive care management. When these infected patients continue to stay in the intensive care unit these multidrug-resistant organisms get opportunity to spread from one patient to another. Soon majority or all the patients in the same unit can get infected with the same multidrug-resistant organism.

So such organisms cause life-threatening infections posing great challenge for treatment for that individual, as well as spread from one patient to another, leading to an outbreak of infection in a unit or hospital. Such organisms can be a great threat to mankind.

Q4. Most of the clinicians know about antibiotic resistance and still continue same practice, why?

There are many reasons, but fear of not curing the patient is foremost. Other reasons are:

- High number of pathogens and complexity of syndromes caused
- Variability over time and place in:
  - Pathogen prevalence
  - Antibiotic susceptibilities
  - Antibiotic formularies
- Poor training in antibiotic use
- Large number and complex drugs
- Availability and cost of microbiological tests
- Parental pressure.

Q5. What is rational or judicial antibiotic practice?

The optimal selection, dose, and duration of an antimicrobial that result in the best clinical outcome for the treatment of infection, with minimal toxicity to the patient and minimal impact on subsequent development of resistance can be called judicial use. The rational use of medicines has been defined by the World Health Organization (WHO) as requiring that patients receive medications appropriate to their clinical needs, in doses that meet their own requirement, for an adequate time, and at the lowest cost to them and their community.

Recently, antimicrobial stewardship is a more frequently used term, which is a combination of antimicrobial management and infection control. It is comprised of:

- Mandatory infection control compliance
- Selection of antimicrobials from each class of drugs that does the least collateral damage
- Appropriate de-escalation when culture results are available.

Q6. What are principles of judicial use of antibiotics?

Basic principles of antibiotic therapy:

- Try to identify the clinical syndrome
- Know the local epidemiology
- Hit fast and as hard as necessary—de-escalate when reports come
- Get the right samples for the lab including for microbiology
- Reassess often.

Q7. What are the criteria for accurate use of antibiotic therapy?

Five criteria of Council for Appropriate and Rational Antibiotic Therapy (CARAT) should be used by clinician described as follows:

1. Evidence-based results
2. Therapeutic benefits
3. Safety
4. Optimal drug for the optimal duration—shorter-course, more aggressive therapy
5. Cost-effectiveness.

Change therapy based on:

- New understanding:
  - Cultures
  - Patient improvement
- Convert to oral and/or narrow spectrum as soon as possible
- Consider alternate diagnoses
  - Do not blindly treat noninfectious syndromes.

Q8. What are the criteria for rational prescription?

We can fit all the important criteria in the word "RATIONALE"

R—Reasoning for prescription, right dose, route, and duration
A—Academically updated decisions
T—Training of mind, residents, parents, and pharmacists
I—Instructions to parents
O—Organism search
N—Noting down the diagnosis
A—Antibiotic policy
L—Local sensitivity pattern
E—Ethical considerations and economic condition of the patient.

Q9. What is appropriate selection of antibiotics for rational use means?

Whatever is an indication, an antimicrobial agent should be the first consideration in choosing appropriate antibiotic therapy. Unambiguous demonstration or the strong suspicion that the etiologic agent is bacterial should only be indication for an antibiotic. This decision should be based on the signs and symptoms of infection, as well as on other factors, including the presence or absence of comorbidities, the patient's medical history, and the age of the patient. If the decision of using antibiotic is finalized, accurate use of the agent should be explored, including examining issues of resistance, benefits, safety, and cost.

For selecting an antibiotic specific guidelines issued by Indian Academy of Pediatrics (IAP) as well as speciality chapters and international groups on the use of antimicrobials for certain infectious diseases should be used. For selecting an antimicrobial agent factors like severity of illness, presence of comorbidities, unusual pathogens, presence of identified clinical risk factors for drug-resistant, and place of therapy (e.g. outpatient versus inhospital) should be taken into account.

In situation where etiologic diagnosis is established or strongly suspected, the antimicrobial agent that is most narrow in spectrum, cost-effective, and least toxic should be used. When one cannot establish etiologic diagnosis empiric antibiotic needs to be selected based on probabilities of pathogen, comorbid conditions, severity of illness, and resistance patterns.

Q10. What do we mean by evidence-based decision in selecting antibiotic which is first principle?

To select the antimicrobial clinical evidence which demonstrates that the antimicrobial agent is clinically and microbiologically appropriate for that infection should be a guide. The well-designed clinical trials should have proved the efficacy of that drug, and the local or region antibiotic resistance patterns for the microbes can help in decision. Professional judgment of clinicians should help to finally choose the optimal antibiotic.

Clinicians can get the highest quality information for making decisions from well-conducted, randomized, and controlled clinical trials by experienced units. Without such information, clinicians may make decisions based on anecdotal experience and traditions which can be wrong in many instances.

Q11. How does issue of therapeutic benefit affect the decision?

Determining the correct diagnosis and analyzing the therapeutic benefits of possible treatments is the key to applying evidence-based results and making appropriate therapeutic choices. To maximize patient health and reduce unnecessary prescribing, each drug should be considered relative to the status of the patient's infection to avail maximum therapeutic benefits. Any evidence that a particular antibiotic can result in a clinical and microbiologic cure, as well as absence of drug treatment can lead to treatment failure, is very important for the clinical decision. The clinician should make all the efforts to identify the causative pathogen and use available data on regional antibiotic resistance patterns in selecting the optimal therapeutic agent.

Data on regional antibiotic resistance patterns help in evaluating available therapeutic choices. To minimize the chances of clinical failure antibacterial susceptibility patterns can be used as guideline though they are based on the results of in vitro tests. So to help proper and rational prescribing practices, data on regional resistance patterns is very important and useful.

Q12. How should one address the safety issues in antibiotic prescriptions?
Safety is most important in treating sick children. Safety must be weighed against efficacy in treating patients with any antimicrobial drug. Although antibiotics are generally considered safe and well tolerated, they have been associated with a wide range of adverse effects. Different classes of antibiotics as well as antibacterial agents within each class have varying degree of safety profile. The safety profiles of newer antimicrobials may not be as well established as those for established agents must be considered before its use.

In the United States, 548 new chemical entities were approved for use in a study period between 1975 and 2000; 16 (2.9%) were withdrawn from the market during this time and 45 of these (8.2%) acquired new black box warnings. One that satisfies all other criteria and has the lowest rate of known adverse events should be selected as antibiotic of choice.

Q13. How should one decide about duration of antibiotic therapy?
Best suited agent to treat the particular infection is an agent from the selected antimicrobial class and the specific member of that class can be called optimal drug. Because empiric therapy is necessary in most cases, multiple factors have to be considered. These factors are—whether the etiologic agent is likely to be gram-positive or gram-negative, the resistance patterns of the likely pathogen to this drug, both nationally and regionally, the individual patient's medical history including recent antibiotic exposure, and whether a narrow or broad-spectrum agent can work. Several professional bodies, such as IAP and the Respiratory Chapter of IAP, have issued guidelines for the use of antimicrobial therapy in community-acquired pneumonia (CAP). The IAP guidelines suggest considering previous health, recent courses of antibiotic treatment, and comorbid conditions for the treatment of outpatients with signs and symptoms of CAP when determining the optimal drug.

Prescribing the selected drug for the shortest amount of time required for clinical and microbiologic efficacy is the *optimal duration*. The potential for reduced occurrence of adverse effects, increased patient adherence, decreased promotion of resistance, and decreased costs are important reasons for reducing antimicrobial therapy to the shortest appropriate duration.

Q14. What is the importance of cost-effectiveness of antibiotics in rational prescription?
Treatment failures and adverse events increase overall cost of medical care which can be a result of choosing inappropriate therapy. In India and internationally, upper respiratory infections including rhinitis, otitis and pharyngotonsillitis, usually mild and nonlife-threatening mostly viral, are

associated with significant health care costs. If hospitalization is required due to treatment failure in outdoor management, results in increased costs. Economic as well as clinical advantages can be achieved by using an optimal course of antibiotics. Children treated optimally in outpatients may return faster to their normal daily routine.

Efficacy of shorter courses of treatment in pneumonia is supported by many studies. For short courses of therapy similar results have also been found for urinary tract infections, bronchitis, and sinusitis.

Q15. Most clinicians think pharmacokinetic considerations are mainly theoretical. Do we need to consider it in rational prescription?

Ability to eradicate bacteria at drug concentrations attained during therapy is a property that can differentiate classes of antibiotics and even among antibiotics within the same class by pharmacokinetic properties. The time for which nonprotein-bound serum concentration of drug exceeds its minimum inhibitory concentration (MIC); the ratio between peak serum concentration (Cmax) and MIC; and the ratio between drug exposure, measured as area under the serum 24-hour concentration-time curve (AUC24), and MIC (AUC24–MIC) ratio are included in these properties. These parameters are very well coordinated with clinical outcome.

For several classes of antibiotics bacteriologic efficacy can be correlated with the time during which drug concentration exceeds MIC, which include the beta-lactams, macrolides, and lincosamides. Thus, these agents should be administered in such way that drug concentrations exceed the MIC for 40% of the dosing interval for optimal reduction of bacterial load. The aminoglycosides, metronidazole, and fluoroquinolones exhibit concentration dependent bactericidal activity in contrast to the time-dependent efficacy of the beta-lactams, macrolides, and lincosamides. The Cmax–MIC and AUC24–MIC ratios correlate with the efficacy of these drugs. Thus, for this class of drug in the absence of adverse effects resulting from high drug doses, administration of a maximum dose for a shorter time would be optimal.

Q16. Are there any simple principles which can guide in rational antibiotic use?

These principles are also termed as golden rules for judicious use of antimicrobials.

Rule 1: Acute infection always presents with fever; in acute illness, absence of fever does not justify antibiotic.

Rule 2: Infection is the most common cause of fever in office practice, though not always bacterial infection.

- Viral infection in majority respiratory tract infection (RTI) especially in children less than 3 years
- Viral infection should not be treated with antibiotic.

Rule 3: Clinical differentiation is possible between bacterial and viral infection most of the times.

- Viral infection is disseminated throughout the system [upper respiratory tract infection/lower respiratory tract infection (URTI/LRTI)].
  - May affect multiple systems
  - Fever is usually high at onset, settles by D3-4
  - Child is comfortable and not sick during inter febrile state
- Bacterial infection is localized to one part of the system (acute tonsillitis does not present with running nose or chest signs)
  - Fever is generally moderate at the onset and peaks by D3-4
- Sneeze and wheeze is nonbacterial unless proved otherwise
- Complete blood count (CBC) does not differentiate between acute bacterial and viral infection.

Rule 4: Chronic infection may not be associated with fever and diagnosis can be difficult

- Relevant laboratory tests are necessary
- Antibiotic is considered only after observing progress
- There is no need to hurry through antibiotic prescription.

Rule 5:

- As far as possible choose single oral antibiotic, either covering suspected gram-positive or negative organism, as per site of infection and age of patient
- Combination of two antibiotics is justified only in serious bacterial infection, without proof of specific organism and may be administered intravenously.

Rule 6:

- At first visit (within 48 hours of fever) antibiotic is justified only if bacterial infection is clinically certain and that does not call for any tests prior to starting the drug (acute tonsillitis/acute otitis media/bacillary dysentery/acute suppurative lymphadenitis)
- If bacterial infection is clinically strongly suspected—should have confirmative tests prior to starting drug, then order relevant tests and start appropriate antibiotic (acute UTI)
- In rest of the cases, in absence of clinical clue and not suspected to have serious disease, observe without antibiotic and follow the progress.

Q17. What are the key interventions to promote rational antibiotics?

- Establishment of a multidisciplinary national body to coordinate policies on medicine use
- Use of clinical guidelines
- Development and use of national essential medicines list
- Establishment of drug and therapeutics committees in districts and hospitals
- Inclusion of problem-based pharmacotherapy training in undergraduate curricula
- Continuing in-service medical education as a licensure requirement
- Supervision, audit, and feedback
- Use of independent information on medicines
- Public education about medicines
- Avoidance of perverse financial incentives
- Use of appropriate and enforced regulation
- Sufficient government expenditure to ensure availability of medicines and staff.

Interventions that promote judicious antibiotic use must be supported by national and local policies. To reduce unnecessary use, National goals should be developed and progress toward those goals should be monitored. To support feedback interventions and program evaluation databases should be established. Economic factors must be carefully considered that may affect practices and modified where necessary.

Surveys of patients' satisfaction or profiling rates of follow-up visits may be an unintended consequence of quality assurance tools, which may lead to antibiotic overuse. To encourage appropriate diagnostic testing, even if this represents a short-term direct cost, support may be needed. Other potential policy options which can help to promote judicious antibiotic use can be sponsorship of continuing education and requirements for renewal of professional licensure.

FURTHER READING

1. Dagan R. What is 'judicious use of antibiotics' and is it achievable in children? Int J Infect Dis. 2014;21(Suppl 1):40-1.
2. Jog P. 'Rationale' of Antibiotic therapy—Think before you ink. Indian Pediatr. 2016;53:775-6.
3. Le Doare K, Barker CI, Irwin A, et al. Improving antibiotic prescribing for children in the resource-poor setting. Br J Clin Pharmacol. 2015;79(3):446-55.
4. Prabhu SV. Judicious antimicrobial therapy in pediatrics, when and what? Pediatr Infect Dis. 2009;1:14-9.
5. WHO. (2011). Frequently asked questions on Antimicrobial resistance. [online] Available from http://apps.who.int/medicinedocs/documents/s19185en/s19185en.pdf [Accessed December, 2018].

CHAPTER 2

Failure of Antibiotic Therapy

Abhay K Shah

Q1. When do we prescribe antibiotic?

Antibiotic is ideally prescribed under following circumstances:

- Proven bacterial infections, as indicated by isolation of an organism in culture or by smear examination
- Near certain bacterial infection e.g. exudative tonsillitis
- Empiric therapy
- Prophylactic use, e.g. urinary tract infection (UTI), rheumatic fever, etc.

Q2. Which are the factors that determine antibiotic response?

Antibiotic response depends on the site of infection, on the pathogen and on the immunological status of the patient.

Although time to response varies for different symptoms and signs, 48–72 hours of adequate therapy are usually needed for improvement in objective signs.

Q3. What are the predictors of antibiotic response?

Response to treatment of an infection can be assessed using clinical, biochemical and microbiological parameters. Sustained defervescence, clinical stability, and improvement of sequential organ function in a 48–72 hours timeframe are the variables that are considered in several studies and seem to better reflect clinical response.

Clinical parameters include improvement in symptoms and signs (e.g. a decrease in fever, tachycardia, respiratory rate, improving sensorium, increasing oral intake, and improving urine output), laboratory values [e.g. decreasing leukocyte count, PCT (procalcitonin) or CRP (C-reactive protein)], organ function markers (reduction or cessation of vasopressors, improvement of hypoxemia among others), and radiologic findings (e.g. improvement in lung opacities). Radiologic improvement can frequently lag behind clinical improvement and routine radiographic follow-up of all infections is not always necessary.

Q4. Which are the common causes for antibiotic failure?

The common causes for antibiotic failure are as under:

- Wrong diagnosis (noninfectious disease)
- Antibiotic-related issues like dose, duration, dosing interval, etc.
- Antibiotic pharmacokinetic and pharmacodynamic (PK/PD) issues
- Development of infectious complication
- Persistence of inflammation
- Inadequate source control
- Antibiotic resistance
- Host immunosuppression.

Q5. Which are common antibiotic factors responsible for antibiotic failure?

- Wrong drug for a wrong bug, e.g. aminoglycosides for *Shigella* and typhoid fever, vancomycin for gram-negative organisms
- *Inadequate dose and incorrect dosing intervals*: This will fail to achieve desirable concentrations in serum and at the site of infections
- *Lack of bactericidal activity*: In presence of bacteremia one should not use bacteriostatic drug, e.g. clindamycin for methicillin-resistant *Staphylococcus aureus* (MRSA) bacteremia
- Poor tissue penetration, e.g. in case of acute bacterial meningitis the antibiotic must penetrate blood-brain barrier. Use of beta-lactam/beta-lactamase inhibitor (BL/BLI) like ceftriaxone-tazobactam and piperacillin-tazobactamis useless.

Q6. Which microbial factors are responsible for antibiotic failure?

- Resistant bacteria, e.g. MRSA, extended-spectrum beta-lactamases (ESBL), and multidrug-resistance (MDR) tuberculosis
- *Anaerobes*: Occult abscesses, secondary subacute bacterial peritonitis, and dental infections. These situations need an appropriate anaerobic coverage
- Polymicrobial infections, e.g. intra-abdominal infections, brain abscess, and neutropenic and immunocompromised patients. These situations need broad spectrum coverage with both aerobic and anaerobic coverage
- *Others*:
  - Viral—needs to be treated with specific antiviral if available
  - Leptospirosis–needs to be diagnosed and treated accordingly
  - Rickettsial disease—needs to be diagnosed
- Fungal—needs antifungal drugs

  It should be suspected in a child with certain risk factors like:
  - Immunocompromised host
  - Neutropenic

- Central venous line
- Receiving antibacterials
- Diabetes mellitus
- Recent corticosteroids.

Q7. What should be our approach in case of antibiotic failure?

Most of the time apparent antibiotic failure results in changing and/or adding a broader spectrum antibiotic, but this will hardly going to be helpful. The most important approach to such antibiotic failure is to analyze the cause of the antibiotic failure by careful evaluation and use of appropriate diagnostic tests to avoid needless, and expensive and potentially dangerous antimicrobial therapy. The important steps would be:

- Maintenance of airway, breathing, circulation, perfusion, nutrition, and euglycemia
- Selection of appropriate antibiotic in correct dose, route, optimum dosing schedule, and duration
- Regular clinical evaluation supported by lab and imaging studies when indicated
- Identification of complication and its remedial measures
- Source control
- Aseptic precautions.

Q8. What is the role of source control in antibiotic failure?

The best recognized example of nonantimicrobial therapy in case of apparent antibiotic failure in the treatment of infections is "source control", namely the use of operative drainage or debridement. This procedure is useful when the organism burden is very high or in the management of abscesses, for which the penetration and activity of antimicrobial agents are often inadequate.

Example: Pleural tapping in complicated pneumonia, removal of subdural fluid in case of acute bacterial meningitis, proper wound care, pus drainage, and debridement of dead tissues in cases of burns, crush injuries, necrotizing fasciitis, etc.

Q9. Which are various mechanisms for antimicrobial resistance?

- Enzymatic degradation of antibacterial drugs, e.g. beta-lactamase and ESBL
- Alteration of bacterial proteins that are antimicrobial targets, e.g. MRSA
- Changes in membrane permeability to antibiotics, e.g. carbapenem-resistance pseudomonas
- Efflux pump, e.g. carbapenem resistance.

Q10. What is the role of antibiotic combination formulations in antibiotic failure/resistance?

For synergistic activity against a microorganism: Synergy between antimicrobial agents means that, when studied in vitro, the combined effect of the agents is greater than the sum of their independent activities when measured separately. For example, the combination of certain beta-lactams and aminoglycosides exhibits synergistic activity against a variety of gram-positive and gram-negative bacteria and is used in the treatment of serious infections, for which rapid killing is essential (e.g. treatment of endocarditis caused by *Enterococcus* species with a combination of penicillin and gentamicin).

In a critically ill patient, empiric therapy before microbiological etiology and/or antimicrobial susceptibility can be determined.

To extend the antimicrobial spectrum for treatment of polymicrobial infections: When infections are thought to be caused by more than one organism, a combination regimen may be preferred because it would extend the antimicrobial spectrum beyond that achieved by a single agent. For example, most intra-abdominal infections are usually caused by multiple organisms with a variety of gram-positive cocci, gram-negative bacilli, and anaerobes.

To prevent emergence of resistance: The emergence of resistant mutants in a bacterial population is generally the result of selective pressure from antimicrobial therapy. Use of combination therapy would provide a better chance that at least one drug will be effective, thereby preventing the resistant mutant population from emerging as the dominant strain and causing therapeutic failure, e.g. artemisinin-based combination therapy (ACT) for malaria and AKT for tuberculosis.

FURTHER READING

1. Bassetti M, Montero JG, Paiva JA. When antibiotic treatment fails. Intensive Care Med. 2018;44(1):73-5.
2. Menendez R, Cavalcanti M, Reyes S, et al. Markers of treatment failure in hospitalised community acquired pneumonia. Thorax. 2008;63(5):447-52.
3. Parthasarathy A. IAP Text Book of Pediatrics, 2nd edition. New Delhi: Jaypee Brothers Medical Publishers (P) Ltd.; 2002.

CHAPTER 3

General Principles in Antibiotic Therapy

Baldev S Prajapati, Rajal B Prajapati

INTRODUCTION

Antibiotics are prescribed for treating bacterial infections. In practice, it amounts to diagnosing bacterial infection reasonably correct to ensure rational use of antibiotics. Once clinician decides to use antibiotics, it is important for him to know clinical application of pharmacokinetics (PK) and pharmacodynamics (PD) of the drug. In recent science, there are ample evidences that application of PK-PD principles to the use of antibiotics results in improved efficacy and decreased the risk of resistance and adverse events.

Q1. What are the principle uses of antibiotics?

- *Therapeutic uses*:
  - *Definitive*: Proven pathogens with or without antibiotic susceptibility available
  - *Empirical*: Bacterial infection most likely but exact organism and sensitivity is not known
  - *Pre-emptive*: Probable bacterial infection on clinical grounds only, waiting for confirmation of bacterial infection may be hazardous, therefore start antibiotics
- *Prophylactic uses*: This should be resorted to only under specific situations. The antibiotic used for prophylaxis should have exquisite activity against the infectious agent even on prolonged use. There should be a significant risk of developing the disease to the host and there should be a justifiable risk ratio.

Q2. What do we mean by PK and PD?

Pharmacokinetics: Kinetics refers to movement. PK deal with drug actions as it moves through the body. Therefore, PK discusses how a drug is:

- Absorbed (taken into body)
- Distributed (moved into various tissues)
- Metabolized (changed into a form that can be excreted)
- Excreted (removal from the body)

- It is also concerned with onset of action of drugs, its peak concentration and duration of action.
  Pharmacokinetics is what the body does to drugs **(Fig. 1)**.

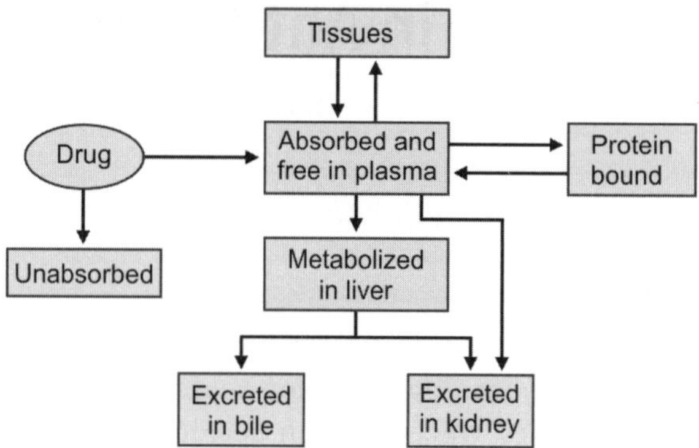

Fig. 1: Pharmacokinetics.

Pharmacodynamics: Pharmacodynamics describes the effect of the drug on the body and the microorganisms **(Fig. 2)**. It is the study of drug mechanisms that produce biochemical changes in the body. The interaction at the cellular level between a drug and cellular components like cell membrane, enzymes or receptors represents the drug action. The response resulting from this drug action is the drug effect.

Pharmacodynamics is what the drugs do to the body.

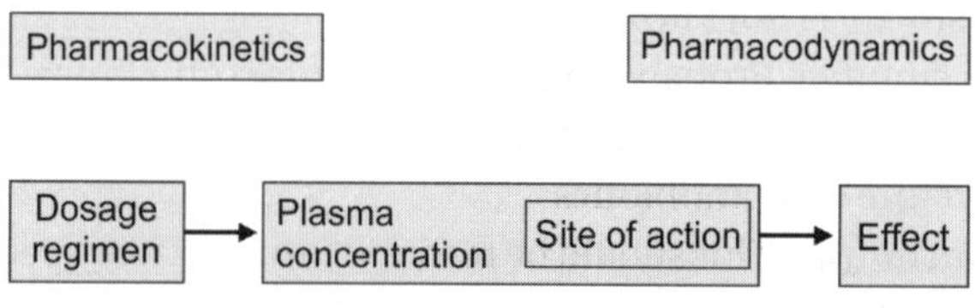

Fig. 2: Pharmacodynamics.

Q3. What should be the preferred route of administration of antibiotics?

- If the patient is stable and able to take orally, tolerating, oral route is preferred.
- Parenteral administration in seriously ill patients where predictable concentration of drug is must like bacterial meningitis, infective endocarditis, neonatal sepsis, etc. Gastrointestinal bleeds, intolerance to oral medications, and adherence issues are other indications for parenteral route.

- Intramuscular route in children and especially in neonates is not preferred due to small muscle mass and erratic absorption. There is also danger of sclerosis and abscess formation due to some irritant drugs.
- Patients with active infections on parenteral antibiotics, once show signs and symptoms of improving clinical status or resolving, can be switched on oral therapy.

Q4. Why oral route for antibiotic therapy in neonates is not recommended?

- *Altered gastric pH*: Alkaline at birth, variable during first month, and approaches to adult value during first 2 years
- Slow or irregular gastric emptying
- Variable and unpredictable intestinal motility
- Gastroesophageal reflux
- Poor pancreatic functions
- Gut colonization and osmotic load may cause diarrhea.

Q5. What are advantages of parenteral to oral switch on therapy?

- Discomfort of intravenous (IV) line is avoided
- Infusion-related adverse events can be avoided
- Reduced cost
- Earlier discharge from hospital.

Q6. What are the types of IV to oral therapy conversions?

- *Sequential therapy*: Replacement of IV drug with oral version of same drug; e.g. linezolid and amoxiclav.
- *Switch therapy*: It is used to describe a conversion from an IV medication to the oral equivalent that may be within the same class and have the level of potency, but is a different compound; e.g. ceftriaxone to cefixime in enteric fever and ceftriaxone to cefpodoxime in pneumonia.
- *Step-down therapy*: It refers to converting from an injectable medication to oral agent in another class or to a different medication within the same class where the frequency, dose and spectrum of activity may not be the same; e.g. vancomycin to clindamycin or linezolid and IV cloxacillin to oral cephalexin in osteomyelitis.

Q7. What are the examples of IV to oral conversion?

- Sequential therapy (same drug is given orally)
- Oral formulations:
  - Azithromycin
  - Ciprofloxacin

- Linezolid
- Metronidazole
- Co-amoxiclav
- Cefuroxime
- Clindamycin
- Switch/step-down therapy

IV drug		Oral drug
• Ampicillin	→	• Amoxicillin
• Ampicillin-sulbactam	→	• Amoxiclav
• Ceftriaxone	→	• Cefixime/cefpodoxime
• Vancomycin	→	• Linezolid
• Cefazolin	→	• Cephalexin
• Cefepime	→	• Ciprofloxacin/levofloxacin

Q8. In which clinical conditions, parenteral to oral switch on therapy is not permitted?

- Neonatal sepsis
- Bacterial meningitis
- Infective endocarditis
- Neutropenia
- Brain abscess
- Orbital cellulitis.

Q9. What factors influence the absorption of various drugs?

- *Absorbed better on empty stomach*:
  - Rifampicin
  - INH
  - Azithromycin
  - Ampicillin
  - Cloxacillin
- *Absorbed better with food*:
  - Cefpodoxime
  - Cefuroxime
  - Nitrofurantoin
- *Factors influencing absorption*:
  - *Fatty meal improves absorption*: Lumefantrine, griseofulvin, and itraconazole
  - *Calcium, magnesium, and antacids lower the absorption*: Tetracyclines and fluoroquinolones.

Q10. What is loading dose of an antibiotic? Is it required? How is it useful?

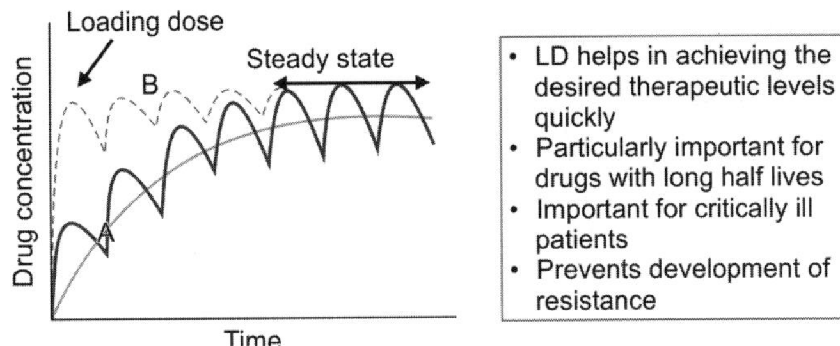

Fig. 3: Loading dose (LD) of an antibiotic.

A loading dose is a first dose of a drug before dropping down to a lower maintenance dose **(Fig. 3)**.

The graph represents the drug accumulation to a steady state without loading dose (A) and with loading dose (B). When a drug is administered, it takes about three to five drug half-lives to reach the therapeutic steady state, i.e. a state when the amount of drug entering the plasma will equal the amount of drug leaving the plasma. Therefore, for an antibiotic with longer plasma half-life like aminoglycosides, if given without loading dose, subtherapeutic drug concentrations will exist for a longer duration, 1–2 days of initial therapy, unless a loading dose is administered. The loading dose will quickly bring the patient's drug concentration to the desired therapeutic concentration.

The recommendations surrounding the need for loading dose were primarily considered only for antibiotics with long half-lives; yet, there is a growing consensus that this may be important even when the drug half-life is short, especially in critically ill patients. Patient's drug exposures within 24 hours of starting therapy may be the most critical period for determining treatment outcome and risk for emergence of multidrug-resistant (MDR) pathogens. This is because the first antibiotic dose is typically administered when inoculums of infection are high and likely to harbor moderately or severely resistant subpopulations. Variable, fluctuating or suboptimal antibiotic concentrations during the first few days of therapy, greatly increases the risk of selecting resistant subpopulations that later breakthrough in the patient with untreatable levels of resistance. If the drug is given without loading dose, it may take care of pathogens which are highly susceptible but not the resistant pathogens which can multiply in subtherapeutic concentrations of antibiotic.

Other examples of drugs for loading dose are aminoglycosides, vancomycin, and chloroquine.

Q11. What do we mean by time-dependent killing antibiotics? How they work in body?

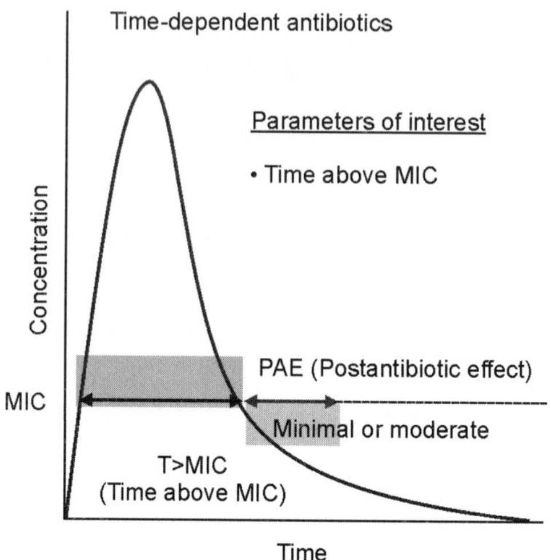

Fig. 4: Time-dependent killing antibiotics. (MIC: minimum inhibitory concentration)

The graph represents time-dependent killing where time the concentration of the drug remains above minimum inhibitory concentration (MIC) (T>MIC) is important **(Fig. 4)**. It should be at least more than 50% of the dosing interval. It has minimal postantibiotic effect; E.g. beta-lactam antibiotics.

Q12. What are concentration-dependent killing antibiotics? What is the mechanism of action?

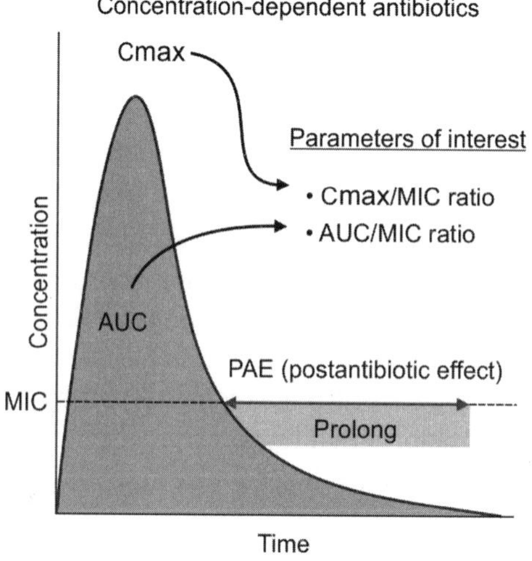

Fig. 5: Concentration-dependent killing antibiotics. (AUC: area under curve; Cmax: peak level of concentration; MIC: minimum inhibitory concentration)

The peak level of concentration (Cmax) is important and it capitalizes on the postantibiotic effect of the drug. Examples: aminoglycosides and fluoroquinolones **(Fig. 5)**.

Q13. What is time-dependent killing with persistent effect?

There is a third type of mode of action. These drugs have both time-dependent killing and concentration-dependent killing. For these drugs, it is the shaded area below the curve (AUC) over the MIC which is important **(Fig. 5)**. Examples: Vancomycin, linezolid, clindamycin, and azithromycin.

Q14. What is the classification of antibiotics based on their PK and PD?

Table 1: Optimal dosing based on PK and PD.

Pattern of activity	*Antimicrobials*	*Optimal dosing based on PK/PD*
Time dependent killing with no persistent effect	Beta lactams	Maximize duration of exposure; T>MIC Use more frequent dosing; longer infusion times including continuous infusion
Concentration-dependent killing with persistent effects	Aminoglycosides, quinilones, daptomycin	Maximize concentrations Cmax > MIC Use less frequent doses and loading dose where possible
Time-dependent killing with persistent effect	Vancomycin Azithromycin Clindamycin	Maximize the AUC/MIC

(AUC: area under curve; Cmax: peak level of concentration; MIC: minimum inhibitory concentration; PD: pharmacodynamic; PK: pharmacokinetic; T>MIC: time above MIC)

It is important to note that once these targets, i.e. T>MIC or peak >MIC or AUC/MIC ratios are achieved there is no evidence that higher ratios result in more rapid killing or less emergence of bacterial resistance, but may on the other hand produce unwanted drug toxicity **(Table 1)**.

Q15. Does pus formation at the site of disease make any difference in effect of antibiotics?

Pus contains phagocytes, cellular debris, and proteins which bind with antibiotics and decreases the penetration of antibiotics at the site of disease. The fluid present in an abscess has low pH, which reduces antimicrobial action, especially of aminoglycosides. Impaired vascular supply into the abscess leads to decreased penetration of antibiotics. In this situation, change of antibiotics is not indicated and good drainage enhances effect of antibiotics.

Q16. Does presence of foreign body make any difference in effect of antibiotics?

Prosthetic material promotes formation of a bacterial biofilm that impairs phagocytosis. Bacterial density is high within the biofilms and bacterial growth is slow. Because rapidly growing organisms are more susceptible to antibiotics than slowly growing, antimicrobial activity is reduced favoring bacterial persistence. Frequent relapses and failure of antibiotics even with long-term and high-dose therapy are common problems with infection in the presence of foreign body. Removal of foreign body enhances effect of antibiotics.

Q17. Which are intracellular pathogens? Which antibiotics are effective with intracellular organisms?

Salmonella, Brucella, Toxoplasma, and *Mycobacterium tuberculosis* are protected from actions of antibiotics that penetrate into the cell poorly.

Macrolides, INH, rifampicin, streptomycin, cotrimoxazole, and fluoroquinolones penetrate cell wall and can achieve intracellular concentration that inhibit or kill pathogens within the cells.

Q18. What is the role of PK and PD in prevention of antimicrobial resistance?

- Optimizing bacterial eradication rates and permitting shorter courses, thereby reducing drug exposure and time depending risk of becoming colonized with resistant pathogens.
- Preventing the emergence of mutational resistance during treatment, where this is known to occur.
- Determining regimens that minimizing resistance risk of transfer resistance between species.
- Determining resistance that minimizes the risk of amplification of important resistant pathogens in normal flora.

Q19. What are PK and PD of antituberculous drugs?

- INH 5 mg/kg/day → Peak level more than 40 MIC
- RMP 10 mg/kg/day → Peak level more than 250 MIC
- RMP is highly lipid soluble and it penetrates well into most of the tissues and is present in effective concentration in all organs and body fluids including cerebrospinal fluid (CSF). It also reaches to caseous foci, phagocytes, etc.

Q20. What is the peculiarity of INH metabolism?

INH is metabolized by acetylation in the liver. There are two types of acetylators; slow and rapid. Rapid acetylators are more prone to hepatotoxicity. Drug dosage is same in both the groups.

Q21. What is effect of different antituberculous drugs on various tuberculous lesions with references to bacterial population (load)?

Table 2: Effects of different antituberculous drugs.

Agent	*Active (extracellular)*	*Semidormant (caseous)*	*Dormant (intracellular)*	*Resistant (mutants)*
INH	+++	++	+	+++
RMP	+++	+++	++	+++
PZA	–	–	+++	–
SM	+++	–	–	+
EMB	++		++	++

- *Group I*:
  - Rapidly multiplying organisms, rapid multiplication is due to neutral pH and oxygen
  - In extracellular environment of pulmonary cavities
  - Best action by INH, RMP, PZA, and SM
- *Group II*:
  - Intermittently multiplying organisms, semidormant, in relatively hypoxic or acid environment of solid caseous material
  - RMP acts very soon after multiplication starts. It acts only during multiplication
- *Group III*:
  - Occasionally dividing organisms, dormant in activated macrophages
  - PZA is most effective
- *Group IV*:
  - Drug-resistant mutants
  - PZA and INH have best action **(Table 2)**.

Q22. What is the basis of multi-agent antituberculous therapy (ATT)?

- Estimated frequency of naturally occurring drug resistant organism is about 10^{-6}.
- Frequency of drug-resistant organism with, SM 10^{-5}, INH 10^{-6}, RMP 10^{-8}, and PZA 10^{-8}.
- Natural occurrence of resistant to one drug is independent of resistance to any other drug.
- The chance that an organism is naturally resistant to both INH and RMP is of 10^{-14}.
- Population of this size does not occur in patients, so least chance of organism naturally resistant to two drugs. This is the basis of multi-agent ATT for active tuberculosis.

- If a patient with extensive pulmonary tuberculosis is given a single medication, sub-population of bacilli susceptible to that drug will be eliminated and resistant subpopulation will multiply and become dormant strain after temporary improvement, resulting in relapse and resistant.

CHAPTER 4

Adverse Effects of Antibiotics and Its Management

Jeeson C Unni, Abhay K Shah

Q1. How will you define adverse effects of antibiotics?

- An antibiotic side (adverse) effect is an unwanted reaction that occurs in addition to the desirable therapeutic action of the antibiotic.
- Antibiotic side effect may interfere with the patient's ability to tolerate and finish the course of medication.

Q2. Which are common factors to be considered for antibiotic side effects?

- Age
- Gender
- Weight
- Body surface area
- Drug interactions
- Genetic predisposition
- Underlying medical disease.

  Such factors might need a dosage and dosing interval modification.

Q3. Which are the common side effects of antibiotics, irrespective of a drug class?

- Gastrointestinal (GI) symptoms: 10%
- Oral thrush
- Vaginal candidiasis
- Pseudomembranous colitis: *Clostridium difficile* and cloxacillin/amoxy
- Phlebitis: Intravenous (IV) use
- Induration: Intramuscular (IM) use
- Allergic reactions: Rash, urticaria, coughing, asthma, and anaphylaxis.

Q4. What are common side effects of penicillins?

Rash, diarrhea, abdominal pain, nausea/vomiting, drug fever, hypersensitivity (allergic) reactions, bronchospasm, vasculitis, serum sickness, exfoliative dermatitis, Stevens-Johnson syndrome, and anaphylaxis. Anaphylaxis and severe skin reaction are an emergency. There is 5–10% cross-sensitivity between penicillin derivatives, cephalosporins, and carbapenems. Reversible biliary sludging is common with third-generation cephalosporins. Renal tubular damage and interstitial nephritis have been associated with large IV doses of penicillin G.

The Jarisch-Herxheimer reaction is a systemic reaction that may occur after the initiation of penicillin therapy and is associated with fever, chills, myalgias, headache, exacerbation of cutaneous lesions, tachycardia, hyperventilation, vasodilation with flushing, and mild hypotension. The pathogenesis of the Herxheimer reaction may be due to the release from the spirochetes of heat-stable pyrogen. There are two types of allergic reactions, i.e. immediate and delayed. Immediate reactions usually occur within 20 minutes of administration and the features vary from urticaria and pruritus to angioneurotic edema, laryngospasm, bronchospasm, hypotension, vascular collapse, and death. Delayed allergic reactions to penicillin therapy usually occur within 1–2 weeks of penicillin therapy. Manifestations include serum sickness-like symptoms, i.e. fever, malaise, urticaria, myalgia, arthralgia, and exfoliative dermatitis.

Penicillin G potassium (1 million units contains 1.7 mEq of potassium ion) may cause serious and even fatal electrolyte disturbances, i.e. hyperkalemia, when given intravenously in large doses.

Ampicillin and cloxacillin may cause pseudomembranous colitis.

Q5. What are common side effects of cephalosporins?

Rash, diarrhea, nausea/vomiting (rare), hypersensitivity (allergic) reactions, serum sickness, vaginal candidiasis, and thrombocytopenia with higher generations of cephalosporins. In conjunction with other nephrotoxic drug it may cause nephrotoxicity. Cross-hypersensitivity may occur in patients with documented penicillin allergy. False positive Coombs test has been reported also occur.

Q6. What are common side effects of aminoglycosides?

Renal toxicity, ototoxicity, dizziness, nausea/vomiting, and nystagmus are common side effects. Out of these, ototoxicity and nephrotoxicity are most important. At time ototoxic damage results in permanent deficit.

Q7. Which are the common factors for aminoglycoside toxicity?

It depends on number of factors.

- Related to the administration of the antibiotic:
  - Previous treatment with aminoglycosides—higher daily doses
  - Prolonged treatment
  - Short dosage intervals
  - Multiple aminoglycoside courses

- Related to characteristics of the patient:
  - Neonates and older patients
  - Dehydration and malnutrition
  - Hypotension and shock
  - Previous renal dysfunction
  - Burns and surgery
  - Liver disease
- Co-administration with other nephrotoxic drugs.

Q8. What is C_{max} and C_{min} in relation to aminoglycosides?

C_{max} refers to the maximum (or peak) serum concentration that a drug achieves after the drug has been administrated and before the administration of a second dose. It mainly deals with efficacy.

C_{min} is the minimum (or trough) concentration that a drug achieves after dosing. It deals mainly with toxicity.

	Nephrotoxicity		*Ototoxicity*	
	C_{max} (µg/mL)	*C_{min} (µg/mL)*	*C_{max} (µg/mL)*	*C_{min} (µg/mL)*
Amikacin	>32–34	>10	>32–34	>10
Tobramycin	>10–12	>2	>10–12	>2
Gentamicin	>10–12	>2	>8	>4

Q9. When to suspect nephrotoxicity?

- Increase in serum creatinine by 50% from base line
- Urinary output less than 0.5 mL/kg/hour for more than 6 hours.

Q10. How will you adjust dose of aminoglycoside in a case of nephrotoxicity?

- First dose as full dose
- Creatinine clearance (CrCl) 51–90: 60–90% 12 hourly
- CrCl 10–50: 30–70% 8–12 hourly
- CrCl less than 10: 20–30% 24–48 hourly
  - CrCl (mL/min) = CrCl(ml/min)= KXL/serum creatinine
  - K is constant 0.5 pediatric
  - .33 for preterm
  - .45 for term baby.

Q11. What are common side effects of carbapenems?

Diarrhea, nausea/vomiting, headache, rash, liver toxicity, and eosinophilia. Local irritation at injection site and pseudomembranous colitis reported rarely. Reversible neutropenia, thrombocytopenia, and thrombocythemia reported. Raised liver enzymes may occur. Adverse central nervous system (CNS) effects such as seizures have been reported particularly in patients with underlying CNS disorders, bacterial meningitis or poor renal function. Drug-related seizures are common with imipenem and hence are not to be used for meningitis. The risk of producing a seizure is more in a child with inadequate dose adjustment in relation to kidney damage. They also cross react with penicillin hypersensitivity.

Q12. What are common side effects of glycopeptides?

- Red man syndrome with rapid (<1 hr) infusion (flushing, hypotension, and itching) and phlebitis. Increasing IV infusion time of vancomycin over 60 minutes may prevent red man syndrome, phlebitis, and rash
- Taste disturbance
- Nausea and vomiting
- Headache and dizziness.
- Foamy urine
- Diarrhea
- Corrected QT (QTc) prolongation
- Nephrotoxicity:
  - Nephrotoxicity; ototoxicity (enhanced by aminoglycoside therapy) but occurs rarely if serum levels are kept below 30 mg/L;
  - Prolonged use more than 3 weeks leads to neutropenia.

Q13. What are common side effects of macrolides?

Minor side effects of macrolides include nausea, vomiting, diarrhea, and ringing or buzzing in the ears (tinnitus). Serious side effects, including allergic reaction and cholestatic hepatitis and are generally associated only with the use of erythromycin. Do not crush, chew, break, open enteric-coated or delayed-release pill.

The most common adverse reactions to erythromycin are GI symptoms, including nausea, vomiting, abdominal cramps, and diarrhea. These side effects are dose-related and result from erythromycin's action on the gastric hormone motilin.

The most common adverse effects reported with azithromycin are diarrhea; nausea; abdominal pain; and headache or dizziness. Laboratory abnormalities include increases in transaminases in 1.5% of patients. Adverse events related to the IV infusion of azithromycin are pain at the injection site and local inflammation (3.1%).

It is recommended that telithromycin be avoided in patients with congenital prolongation of the QTc interval; in those with ongoing proarrhythmic conditions, such as uncorrected hypokalemia or clinically significant bradycardia.

Treatment of young infants with macrolide antibiotics was strongly associated with infantile hypertrophic pyloric stenosis (IHPS) and should therefore only be administered if potential treatment benefits outweigh the risk. Maternal use of macrolides during the first 2 weeks after birth was also associated with an increased risk of IHPS.

Q14. What are common side effects of sulfonamides?

- Nausea/vomiting, diarrhea, anorexia, and abdominal pain
- Skin rash
- Pancytopenias
- Hemolysis in glucose-6-phosphate dehydrogenase (G6PD) deficiency
- Drug fever
- Aseptic meningitis
- photosensitivity, headache, and dizziness
- Serum sickness
- Serious side effects include Stevens–Johnson syndrome, toxic epidermal necrolysis, and drug rash with eosinophilia and systemic symptoms (DRESS) syndrome
- Use of sulfa drugs in a child with G6PD deficiency worsens the course of rickettsial infections.

Q15. What are common side effects of tetracyclines?

Nausea/vomiting, diarrhea, anorexia, abdominal pain, photosensitivity, tooth discoloration in children less than 8 years, and liver toxicity are common side effects of tetracyclines. It may cause linear growth impairment. Avoid prolonged sunlight exposure; use sunscreen, wear protective clothing.

Q16. What are common side effects of quinolones?

The most frequent side effects are GI reactions (nausea, dyspepsia, and vomiting) and CNS reactions such as dizziness, insomnia, and headache. Phototoxicity has been reported in varying frequencies with the different fluoroquinolones, especially with pefloxacin. It can cause seizures, psychosis, and pseudotumor cerebri. Ciprofloxacin, ofloxacin, and pefloxacin were the quinolones with more neurological and psychiatric side effects as reported in the literature. The finding in juvenile animals of cartilage damage after administration of high doses has resulted in recommendations that fluoroquinolones should not be used in children. Moxifloxacin is associated with higher rates of non-neurological side effects. These drugs are not recommended for use in children, years or in pregnant or lactating women. Avoid prolonged sunlight exposure; use sunscreen, and wear protective clothing when photosensitivity is severe.

Q17. What are common side effects of lincomycin derivatives?

- Nausea
- Vomiting
- Swollen or painful tongue
- Vaginal-itching or discharge
- Mild itching or skin rash
- Ringing in your ears
- Dizziness
- Spinning feeling
- Diarrhea
- Hives
- Anal itching
- Hypersensitivity reactions (skin swelling and anaphylaxis)
- Pseudomembranous colitis (may be severe), diarrhea, nausea/vomiting, rash, hypersensitivity, and jaundice (clindamycin)
- If severe diarrhea during treatment or for up to 8 weeks after treatment—pseudomembranous colitis (*C. difficile*); consider use of less toxic agents.

Q18. What are the side effects with antistaphylococcal agents?

Drug	*Side effects*	*Serious*
Cloxacillin	Rash and diarrhea	Pseudomembranous colitis
Clindamycin	Nausea, vomiting, diarrhea, and serum sickness	Pseudomembranous colitis
Vancomycin	Phlebitis and red man syndrome	Ototoxicity and nephrotoxicity
Linezolid	Thrombocytopenia and neutropenia	Peripheral neuropathy
Daptomycin	Myalgia, muscle cramps, and elevated creatine phosphokinase (CPK)	
Quinupristin-Dalfopristin	Pain at infusion site, myalgia, and pruritis	

Q19. What are common side effects of metronidazole?

Nausea/vomiting, dizziness, headache, vaginal candidiasis, and metallic taste are common side effects.

Q20. What are the nephrotoxic antibiotics?

Aminoglycosides such as tobramycin and gentamycin can cause toxicity in "renal tubular cells". In addition to their direct effect on cells, aminoglycosides cause renal vasoconstriction. Aminoglycoside uptake by the tubules is a saturable phenomenon, so uptake is limited after a single dose. Thus, a single daily large dose is preferable to three doses per day. One dose per day presumably causes less accumulation in the tubular cells once the saturation point is reached. Extending the dose interval to more than 24 hours in patients with renal impairment has been found effective, with irreversible nephrotoxicity reported in approximately 1% of the patients studied.

Sulfonamides, as they are weak acids, sulfonamides crystallize in sufficiently acidic urine (pH ≤ 5.5), causing intratubular obstruction and acute decline in renal function. Patients receiving high doses of sulfonamide to treat opportunistic infections are prone to acute kidney injury from crystalluria.

Vancomycin can cause kidney damage due to a combination of the oxidative effects on the proximal renal tubule resulting in renal tubular ischemia and allergic interstitial nephritis.

Q21. What are the hepatotoxic antibiotics?

Amoxicillin/clavulanate and cotrimoxazole, as well as flucloxacillin, cause hepatotoxic reactions (cases are often isolated, may have a delayed onset, sometimes appear only after cessation of therapy and can produce an array of hepatic lesions that mirror hepatobiliary disease, making causality often difficult to establish).

Hepatotoxic reactions related to macrolides, tetracyclines, and fluoroquinolones (in that order, from high to low) are much rarer.

Antibiotics specifically used for tuberculosis—adverse effects range from asymptomatic increases in liver enzymes to acute hepatitis and fulminant hepatic failure.

Q22. What are the antibiotics that cause Stevens–Johnson syndrome?

Trimethoprim/sulfamethoxazole, ceftriaxone, cephalexin, vancomycin, amoxicillin, cloxacillin piperacillin and tazobactam, ciprofloxacin, doxycycline, and clarithromycin are the antibiotics that cause Stevens–Johnson syndrome.

Q23. What are the neurological side effects of antibiotics?

Aminoglycosides have been known to cause ototoxicity most commonly, though peripheral neuropathy, encephalopathy, and neuromuscular blockade have also been reported.

- *Cephalosporins*: Neurotoxicity has been reported with first-generation cephalosporins such as cefazolin, second-generation such as cefuroxime, third-generation such as ceftazidime, and fourth-generation such as cefepime and can range from encephalopathy to nonconvulsive status epilepticus (NCSE)—tardive seizures, encephalopathy, myoclonus, truncal asterixis, seizures, NCSE, and coma.
- Penicillins can also cause neurologic side effects and it include a wide spectrum of manifestations including encephalopathy, behavioral changes, myoclonus, seizures, etc.

- Carbapenems are reported to be associated with seizures with an estimated incidence of 3%.
- Tetracyclines have been associated with cranial nerve toxicity and neuromuscular blockage and benign intracranial hypertension.
- Trimethoprim/sulfamethoxazole has been reported to be associated with encephalopathy and psychosis.
- Macrolides have been linked to ototoxicity via damage to the cochlea.
- Neurotoxic manifestations associated with quinolones include seizures, confusion/encephalopathy, myoclonus, and toxic psychosis. Complex partial status epilepticus or NCSE documented by electroencephalogram (EEG) have been reported with ciprofloxacin-induced neurotoxicity in patients presenting with altered mental status or confusion.
- Polymyxins: Paresthesias and ataxia, and less commonly, diplopia, ptosis and nystagmus.
- Metronidazole can have cerebellar toxicity that manifests clinically with varying degrees of limb and gait ataxia and dysarthria.
- Nitrofurantoin when used in children is associated with a sensorimotor polyneuropathy.
- Minocycline, nalidixic acid, and nitrofurantoin can cause benign intracranial hypertension.

Q24. What are the cardiac side effects of antibiotics?

Underlying risk of arrhythmia is associated with the use of macrolides and fluoroquinolones antibiotics. Torsades de pointes (TdP) is a rare potential side effect of fluoroquinolones and macrolide antibiotics. TdP is a specific type of abnormal heart rhythm that can lead to sudden cardiac death. Prolongation of the QT interval can increase a person's risk of developing this abnormal heart rhythm.

Q25. How to prevent adverse antibiotic reactions?

- Avoid inappropriate use of antibiotics
- Take care of dose, duration, interval, and administrations
- Review of simultaneously used drugs
- Elicit history of allergic diseases and drug allergy
  - A drug responsible for an allergic reaction should not be reused, unless it is an absolutely needed and alternative drug is not available
  - Pretreatment with H1 antihistamines should not be used as they do not prevent anaphylactic shock and may mask early signs
- Serial clinical assessment/laboratory monitoring are crucial
- Avoid detrimental combinations

- Learn the art of de-escalation
- Drug level monitoring: Aminoglycosides and vancomycin
- Skin prick tests may be helpful for diagnosing immunoglobulin E (IgE) dependent drug reactions
- Radioimmunoassays [like radioallergosorbent test (RAST)] may detect serum IgE antibodies to certain drugs (penicillin)
- Oral provocation tests: They must be performed under strict medical supervision with resuscitative equipment available. Although seldom required, they may be regarded as the "gold standard".

CHAPTER 5

Chemoprophylaxis

Janani Sankar

Q1. What do you understand by chemoprophylaxis?

Antibiotics have been used prophylactically to:

- Prevent infections by giving the drug before or soon after the acquisition of an inoculating organism
- Prevent a resident organism from infecting a normally sterile site
- Prevent a dormant pathogenic organism from causing disease.

Q2. What are the prerequisites while choosing a chemoprophylactic drug?

For prophylaxis to be effective the nature of the invading organism must be predictable and an antibiotic specific to that particular organism should be chosen. The antibiotic should be safe for long-term use and usually it is a long acting drug.

Q3. What are types of antimicrobial prophylaxis?

Antimicrobial prophylaxis may be considered primary (prevention of an initial infection) or secondary (prevention of the recurrence or reactivation of an infection), or it may also be administered to prevent infection by eliminating a colonizing organism

Q4. What are the contexts where chemoprophylaxis is advised?

The contexts where chemoprophylaxis is given are:

1. For close contacts of patients with infections which spread through droplets to prevent infection in contacts.
2. For patients themselves to prevent specific infections depending on their underlying condition, e.g. anatomical abnormality of genitourinary system such as PUV, primary immune deficiency, etc.

Q5. What are the indications for contact chemoprophylaxis?

Infections requiring chemoprophylaxis for contacts:

1. Diphtheria

Erythromycin—40 mg/kg/day for 7–10 days or single IM dose of Benzathine

Penicillin (0.6 mega units for < 30 kg body weight and 1.2 mega units for > 30 kg body weight).

2. Pertussis

Erythromycin 40–50 mg/kg/day in four divided doses for 14 days.

3. Neisseria meningitis

Antimicrobial prophylaxis for meningococcal diseases should be offered to close contacts of sporadic cases of *Neisseria meningitidis* infection. Close contacts include household members, day care center staff, and any person directly exposed to an infected person's oral secretions. Given to close contacts to eliminate nasopharyngeal carriage preferably within 24 hours of contact with an index case.

- Ciprofloxacin is the drug of choice 15 mg/kg—single oral dose
- Ceftriaxone—125 mg IM for children < 12 years, 250 mg> 12 years
- Rifampicin 10 mg/kg Q12H, a total of four doses

4. Plague

Close contact with a patient infected with pneumonic plague should be kept under surveillance for atleast 1 week. The drugs used for chemoprophylaxis of close contacts are Ciprofloxacin 20 mg/kg/day in two divided doses. Doxycycline can also be used.

5. Mycobacterium tuberculosis

According to recent RNTCP recommendations any child less than 6 years of age who is in close contact with an open case of Tuberculosis should receive Isoniazid Preventive Therapy (IPT) 10 mg/kg/day for 6 months after excluding active disease irrespective of the child's BCG or nutritional status.

It is also recommended for all HIV infected children, children who are TST positive and on immunosuppressive therapy, child born to a mother who was treated for tuberculosis in the antenatal period after ruling out congenital tuberculosis.

6. Varicella

Oral Acyclovir 200 mg/day for immunosuppressed patients and post-transplant patients who have contact with varicella patients.

7. H1N1 infection

The following patients who are in contact with H1NI positive patients need prophylaxis with Oseltamivir

- Infants 3–12 months: 3 mg/kg/day for 10 days
- High risk children less than 12 kg: 35 mg/day for 10 days
  - 12–23 kg: 45 mg/day for 10 days
  - 23–40 kg: 60 mg/day for 10 days
  - More than 40 kg: 75 mg/day for 10 days.

Q.6. How do we prevent malaria in overseas travelers traveling to malarial endemic areas?

Travelers traveling to malarial endemic areas are advised to follow either of the following regimen:

- *Short-term up to 6 weeks*: Doxycycline 1.5 mg/kg once a day for children above 8 years—maximum dose 100 mg. Ideal to start 2 days before arrival and continue for 4 weeks after leaving the endemic area.
- *Long-term more than 6 weeks*: Mefloquine 5 mg /kg (up to 250 mg) weekly started 2 weeks before and 4 weeks after leaving the endemic area.

Q.7. What are the conditions where chemoprophylaxis is advised for patients?

Conditions requiring chemoprophylaxis for patients:

1. Urinary tract infections:

Indications and duration of prophylaxis: The indications and duration of prophylaxis depend on patient age and presence or absence of VUR. Antibiotic prophylaxis is recommended for patients with—(i) UTI below 1 year of age, while awaiting imaging studies, (ii) VUR, (iii) frequent febrile UTI (three or more episodes in a year) even if the urinary tract is normal. Antibiotic prophylaxis is not advised in patients with urinary tract obstruction (e.g. posterior urethral valves), urolithiasis and neurogenic bladder, and in patients on clean intermittent catheterization Children with VUR and recurrent UTI and those with anatomical

- For VUR, Grades I and II antibiotic prophylaxis until 1-year-old. Restart antibiotic prophylaxis if breakthrough febrile UTI.
- Grades III to V—antibiotic prophylaxis up to 5 year of age. Consider surgery if breakthrough febrile UTI. Antibiotic prophylaxis is continued for 6 months after surgical repair.
- Beyond 5 year: Prophylaxis continued if there is bowel bladder dysfunction.

The options are antimicrobials for prophylaxis of urinary tract infections—

- Cotrimoxazole 1–2 dose, mg/kg/day as trimethoprim dose
  Avoid in infants <3 Months, G6PD deficiency
- Cephalexin (10 mg/kg/day)
- Nitrofurantoin (1–2 mg/kg/day), avoid in infants < 3 months, G6PD deficiency, renal insufficiency

2. Acute rheumatic fever:

Penicillin G: IM 600,000 units every 21–28 days

or

Penicillin V 250 mg orally twice a day

In case of Penicillin allergy—erythromycin 20 mg/kg/dose twice daily or azithromycin 5 mg/kg orally once a day—maximum 250 mg/day. The duration of prophylaxis varies based on the risk of recurrence and severity of disease.

Antimicrobial prophylaxis should be considered lifelong or at least until age 40 years (whichever is longer) for patients with severe carditis with persistent valvular disease. Prophylaxis should be continued in patients even after prosthetic valve replacement surgery.

For patient with rheumatic fever with carditis without valvular damage it should be given for 10 years or till 25 years of age, whichever is longer. Rheumatic fever with no carditis for 5 years

3. Infective endocarditis:

Children with the conditions mentioned below should receive chemoprophylaxis 30–60 minutes before dental procedure.

1. Prosthetic material used for cardiac valve repair, such as annuloplasty rings and chords.
2. Previous IE.
3. Unrepaired cyanotic congenital heart disease or repaired congenital heart disease, with residual shunts or valvular regurgitation at the site of or adjacent to the site of a prosthetic patch or prosthetic device.
4. Cardiac transplant with valve regurgitation due to a structurally abnormal valve.

The drugs that can be used are amoxicillin 50 mg/kg. If allergic to penicillin Azithromycin 15 mg/kg or Clindamycin 20 mg/kg or Cephalexin 50 mg/kg.

4. Asplenia/sickle cell disease/post-splenectomy:

For children who are at higher risk for severe infections based on young age, concurrent immunocompromising conditions or history of sepsis caused by encapsulated bacteria. Daily antibiotic prophylaxis till 18 years of age or for life.

5. Asplenia/splenectomy:

The duration is until 5 years of age or atleast 1 year following splenectomy.

- Preferred agents: Penicillin V < 3 years 125 mg orally twice a day >3 years 250 mg orally twice a day.
- Alternative agents:
  - Amoxicillin 10 mg/kg orally twice daily
  - Cephalexin 25 mg/kg orally twice daily
  - Azithromycin 5 mg/kg once a day (maximum 500 mg/dose)

During febrile episodes

- Amoxicillin clavulanate 45 mg/kg orally twice a day

- Cefuroxime 15 mg/kg orally twice daily
- Levofloxacin 10 mg/kg twice daily

6. Primary immune deficiency:

1. Patients with SCID or other combined immune deficiency—combination of antibacterial, antiviral and or antifungal prophylaxis
2. Patients with CGD—prophylactic antibiotics, antifungal and interferon gamma
3. Patients with NK cell deficiency syndrome—antiviral prophylaxis
4. Patients with MSMD (Mendelian Susceptibility to Mycobacterial Diseases) require prophylaxis against mycobacterial infections

Antibiotic options include:

- Amoxicillin: 10–20 mg/kg/day as a single dose or twice daily dose
- Trimethoprim: Sulfamethoxazole 5 mg/kg/day of trimethoprim as a single dose or twice daily
- Azithromycin: 10 mg/kg/week or 5 mg/kg every other day.

Q.8. What are the current recommendations for prevention of surgical site infections?

Surgical site infections:

1. *Clean wounds:* Uninfected operative wounds where no inflammation is present and there is no entry into respiratory, GIT or genitourinary tracts and hence there is no need for prophylaxis.
2. *Clean contaminated wounds*: The respiratory, alimentary and genitourinary tracts are entered under controlled conditions with no significant risk of contamination. Prophylaxis is indicated in procedures where a substantial amount of wound contamination is expected.
3. *Contaminated wounds:* This includes open wounds, accidental wounds, penetrating wounds, and infections where acute inflammation is expected.
4. *Dirty and infected wounds:* Penetrating wounds of more than 4 hours duration, perforated viscera, and wounds with inflammation.

Recommendations for preoperative antimicrobial prophylaxis operation.

Preoperative dose

Neonatal (≤72 hr of age):

All major procedures group B streptococci, enteric gram-negative bacilli, enterococci, coagulase-negative staphylococci—

Ampicillin 50 mg/kg
plus
Gentamicin 4 mg/kg

Neonatal (>72 hr of age):
All major procedures prophylaxis targeted to colonizing organisms, nosocomial organisms.

Cardiac (cardiac surgical procedures, prosthetic valve or pacemaker, ventricular assist devices)
Staphylococcus epidermidis, Staphylococcus aureus, Corynebacterium species, enteric gram-negative bacilli Cefazolin *or* (if MRSA or MRSE is likely) Vancomycin 30 mg/kg (maximum 2 g) 15 mg/kg.

Gastrointestinal

- Esophageal and gastroduodenal enteric gram-negative bacilli, a gram-positive cocci
- Cefazolin (high risk only b) 30 mg/kg (maximum 2 g)
- Biliary tract enteric gram-negative bacilli, a enterococci
- Cefazolin 30 mg/kg (maximum 2 g).

Colorectal or appendectomy (uncomplicated, nonperforated)/enteric gram-negative bacilli, a enterococci, anaerobes (Bacteroides species)
Cefoxitin 40 mg/kg (maximum 3 g)
With or without Gentamicin 2.5 mg/kg
or
Gentamycin 2.5 mg/kg
plus
Metronidazole 15 mg/kg
plus
Ampicillin 50 mg/kg
or
Meropenem 20 mg/kg

Genitourinary enteric gram-negative bacilli, enterococci
Cefazolin 30 mg/kg (maximum 2 g)
or
Ampicillin 50 mg/kg (maximum 2 g)
plus
Gentamicin 2.5 mg/kg

Head and neck surgery (incision through oral or pharyngeal mucosa) anaerobes, enteric gram-negative bacilli, *S. aureus*
Clindamycin 10 mg/kg (maximum 600 mg)
With or without Gentamicin 2.5 mg/kg
or
Cefazolin 30 mg/kg (maximum 2 g)
plus
Metronidazole 15 mg/kg (maximum 1 g)

Neurosurgery (craniotomy, intrathecal baclofen shunt or ventricular shunt placement) *S. epidermidis, S. aureus*
Cefazolin
or
(if MRSA or MRSE is likely) Vancomycin 30 mg/kg (maximum 2 g) 15 mg/kg.

Q.9. What are measures to prevent recurrent pustulosis?
Recurrent pyogenic skin infections caused by *Staphylococcus aureus*, including methicillin-resistant *S. aureus* (MRSA), may be managed by encouraging good personal hygiene, the avoidance of shared personal items, and the diligent cleaning of high-touch environmental surfaces. If a patient is found to be colonized by *S. aureus*, nasal decolonization with mupirocin for 5–10 days with or without a topical body decolonization with a skin antiseptic solution such as 4% chlorhexidine for 5–14 days may be reasonable in an attempt to decolonize the patient.

FURTHER READING

1. AAP. Red Book 2018-21, 31st edition. Illinois: American Academy of Pediatrics; 2018.
2. Consensus guidelines on Pediatric Rheumatic fever. Indian Pediatr. 2008;45:565-73.
3. Gupta P. PG Textbook of Pediatrics, 2nd edition. New Delhi: Jaypee Brothers Medical Publishers (P) Ltd.; 2015.
4. Indian Nephrology Society Group. Recommendations for UTI. Gurugram: INSG; 2015.
5. Kliegman RM, Stanton B, Geme JS, et al. Nelson Text Book of Pediatrics, 20th edition. New Delhi: Elsevier; 2015.

SECTION 2

Common Infections in Office Practice

- Tonsillopharyngitis
- Diphtheria
- Otitis Media: Acute, Recurrent
- Sinusitis
- Whooping Cough
- Community-acquired Pneumonias
- Empyema
- Suppurative Lung Diseases
- Acute Diarrheal Disorders
- Urinary Tract Infection
- Enteric Fever
- Spontaneous Bacterial Peritonitis
- Skin and Soft Tissue Infections and Necrotizing Fasciitis
- Septic Arthritis
- Osteomyelitis
- Acute Bacterial Meningitis
- Brain Abscess
- Ring Lesions

CHAPTER 6

Tonsillopharyngitis

Jaydeep Choudhury

Q1. What are the causes of acute tonsillopharyngitis?

Viruses are the usual causes. Important viruses that cause tonsillopharyngitis are influenza, parainfluenza, adenovirus, coronavirus, enterovirus, rhinovirus, respiratory syncytial virus, etc. Group A *Streptococcus* (*Streptococcus pyogenes*) is the most common bacterial cause. Other bacteria like Arcanobacterium, Francisella, *Mycoplasma, Chlamydia, Fusobacterium* and *Corynebacterium* may also cause tonsillopharyngitis.

Q2. What are the characteristic features for strep throat?

Common signs and symptoms of streptococcal pharyngitis include sore throat, temperature greater than 100.4°F (38°C), tonsillar exudates, and cervical adenopathy. Cough, coryza and diarrhea are more common with viral pharyngitis.

Q3. How to establish bacterial cause of pharyngitis?

Clinically, it is difficult to distinguish as the symptoms and signs overlap. Streptococcal pharyngitis is uncommon before 2 years of age. It is more common in 5–15 years age group.

Throat swab culture and rapid antigen detection tests (RADTs) are the diagnostic tests for Group A *Streptococcus* (GAS). Throat swab culture remains the gold standard. RADTs have high specificity hence it can also be used for diagnosis of GAS. Most of the time strep throat remains a clinical diagnosis.

Q4. What is the treatment for acute tonsillopharyngitis?

Symptomatic treatment is the main treatment plan for acute tonsillopharyngitis, as most of the infections are due to viruses. Oral antipyretics or analgesics like paracetamol are the mainstay of symptomatic treatment along with maintaining hydration and nutrition.

Q5. When should presumptive antibiotic be started?

Presumptive antibiotic should be started in the following situations, but a confirmatory test should be performed:

- When there is a clinical diagnosis of scarlet fever
- Symptomatic child with household contact with a documented GAS pharyngitis
- History of acute rheumatic fever in the patient or a family member.

Q6. What happens if GAS pharyngitis is not treated?

If antibiotic is started within 48 hr of the onset of the illness, it reduces the duration and severity of symptoms, as well as the risk of local complications and the likelihood that infection will spread to others.

Most untreated GAS pharyngitis resolves within 5 days. The intent of antibiotic therapy is the prevention of acute rheumatic fever. It is effective even if treatment is started as late as 9 days of onset of illness. Antibiotic therapy does not prevent acute poststreptococcal glomerulonephritis.

Q7. What antibiotics are used for treating acute streptococcal pharyngotonsillitis?

Amoxicillin is the drug of choice. The dose is 40 mg/kg/day in 2 or 3 divided doses orally for 10 days. Alternately, Cephalexin or Cefadroxil (first generation cephalosporins) may be used orally for 10 days. Macrolides may be used in penicillin allergic patients. Clarithromycin 15 mg/kg/day for 10 days in 2 divided doses or Azithromycin 12 mg/kg on day 1 and then, 6 mg/kg from day 2 to 5.

Q8. How will you manage recurrent tonsillitis?

Recurrent sore throat are quite common in our day to day practice. Majority of them are viral and children may have 4 to 6 such episodes in a year. However, classical recurrent strep throat is not that commo. Many times there seems to be overdiagnosis. This has to be confirmed by throat cultures (the gold standard) or rapid strep detection tests. Rapid strep detection tests improve the accuracy of diagnosing strep throat infections. However positive results must be differentiated from carrier and true clinical infection. Commonest cause of failure is incomplete course of prescribed antibiotic. Strep throat infections are often now a days resistant to Erythromycin, and azithromycin . Even when all strep infections are laboratory confirmed with throat cultures or rapid strep detection tests, and the antibiotic is finished, failure to respond to treatment still occurs. Patients who do not respond to penicillin or amoxicillin treatment failure are those who have recently received treatment with these drugs and are then retreated with the same antibiotic.The antibiotic options in such cases are Oral first generation cephalosporins or amoxiclav or clindamycin . When Cephalosporin are used to treat strep throat infections, a failure occurs less than 5% of the time; however, they are more expensive than penicillin or amoxicillin.Amoxicillin/clavulanic acid has been shown to be superior or equivalent in comparison to penicillin. Clindamycin or rifampin, in combination with a second antibiotic, such as penicillin, amoxicillin, or a cephalosporin, has been used to treat acute, recurrent, and carrier strep throat infections. However rifampicin is to be spared only for tuberculosis.

If a patient has six to seven recurrent strep throat infections over a one-to two-year time span, then a tonsillectomy should be considered. However, the risk of surgery and anesthesia should be weighed against the discomfort and sufferings caused by recurrent tonsillitis.

CHAPTER 7

Diphtheria

Jaydeep Choudhury

Q1. What are the diagnostic modalities of diphtheria?

Diagnosis of diphtheria is mainly clinical. Swab culture is the gold standard for diagnosis of diphtheria. Specimens for culture should be obtained from the throat and nose and also from any other mucocutaneous lesion. Ideally a portion of the membrane with exudates should be cultured. Isolation of *Corynebacterium diphtheriae* requires special culture media containing tellurite agar or especially enriched Loeffler, Hoyle, Mueller, or Tinsdale medium.

Evaluation of a direct smear using Gram stain or Albert stain or specific fluorescent antibody is unreliable and hence not indicated. Diagnostic tests used to confirm diphtheria infection combine isolation of *C. diphtheriae* on cultures with toxigenicity testing. The later can be performed using the Elek test. But it is not readily available in most of the clinical microbiology laboratories. Polymerase chain reaction (PCR) test may be done.

Q2. What are the various supportive cares of diphtheria?

Bed rest is essential during the acute phase of illness which is usually for 2 weeks or until the risk for symptomatic cardiac damage has passed. Return to physical activity is guided by the degree of toxicity and cardiac involvement. Droplet precautions are required till cessation of therapy or culture negativity. Cutaneous wounds are cleaned thoroughly with soap and water. Diphtheritic membrane in throat and peripharyngeal edema may cause airway obstruction. Mechanical ventilation may be required under such circumstances. Complications like myocarditis or palatal palsy or neuropathy may require critical care management.

Q3. What are the specific antitoxins?

Antitoxins for diphtheria are the mainstay of therapy and should be administered on the basis of clinical diagnosis. Antitoxins should be administered at the earliest. The main reason is that it neutralizes only free toxin. The efficacy of antitoxin diminishes with time elapsed after the onset of mucocutaneous symptoms. Diphtheria antitoxin is administered as a single empirical dose of 20,000–120,000 U based on the degree of toxicity, site and size of the membrane, and duration of illness. Antitoxin is probably of no value for local manifestations of cutaneous diphtheria, but its use is prudent because of the possibility of toxic sequelae. Commercially available intravenous (IV) immunoglobulin preparations is not proven or approved for therapy of diphtheria because it contains low titers of antibodies to diphtheria toxin. Antitoxin is not recommended for asymptomatic carriers.

Q4. What are the antimicrobial therapies of diphtheria?

The most effective antibiotics for diphtheria are penicillins or erythromycins. The utility of antibiotics is mainly because it decreases or stops toxin production, treats localized infection and prevent transmission of the organism to contacts. Only penicillin or erythromycin is recommended for treatment. Erythromycin is marginally superior to penicillin for eradication of nasopharyngeal carriage. Appropriate therapy is erythromycin (40–50 mg/kg/day divided every 6 hr by mouth or IV; maximum 2 g/day), aqueous crystalline penicillin G [100,000–150,000 U/kg/day divided every 6 hr IV or intramuscular (IM)], or procaine penicillin (25,000–50,000 U/kg/day divided every 12 hr IM) for 14 days. Treatment with erythromycin is repeated if either culture yields *C. diphtheriae* after completion of therapy.

Q5. How to manage household contacts?

All the household contacts and others who had intimate respiratory or habitual physical contact with a patient suffering from diphtheria are closely monitored for illness through the 7 day incubation period of *C. diphtheriae.* Cultures of nose, throat, and any cutaneous lesions should be performed. Antimicrobial prophylaxis is presumed effective and is administered regardless of immunization status, using erythromycin (40–50 mg/kg/day divided qid PO for 10 days; maximum 2 g/day) or a single injection of benzathine penicillin G (600,000 U IM for patients <30 kg, 1,200,000 U IM for patients ≥ 30 kg). Diphtheria toxoid vaccine, in age-appropriate form, is given to immunized individuals who have not received a booster dose within last 5 years. Children who have not received their fourth dose diptheria, tetanus toxoids, and pertussis (DTP) vaccine should be vaccinated. Those who have received fewer than three doses of diphtheria toxoid or who have uncertain immunization status are immunized with an age-appropriate primary schedule of diphtheria vaccine.

Q6. How to follow-up a child after treatment?

Repeat cultures are performed after a minimum of 2 weeks following completion of therapy in patients and carriers. If the results are positive, an additional 10 days course of oral erythromycin should be administered and follow-up cultures performed.

Q7. How the carrier state is managed?

The following steps are initiated when an asymptomatic carrier is identified. Antimicrobial prophylaxis is administered for 7–10 days. An age-appropriate preparation of diphtheria toxoid is immediately administered if the patient has not received a booster injection within last 1 year. Individuals are placed in strict isolation (respiratory tract colonization) or contact isolation (cutaneous colonization only) until at least two subsequent cultures taken 24 hours apart after cessation of therapy demonstrate negative results.

Q8. What should be the vaccination strategy in a patient suffering from diphtheria?

Diphtheria disease might not confer immunity to the individual. Persons recovering from diphtheria should begin or complete active immunization with diphtheria toxoid containing vaccines during convalescence. Children should receive active immunization as per schedule 6 weeks after the acute illness.

FURTHER READING

1. John TJ. Resurgence of diphtheria in India in the 21st century. Indian J Med Res. 2008;128:669-70.
2. Nath B, Mahanta TG. Investigation of an outbreak in Borborooah block of Dirbrugarh district, Assam. Indian J Community Med. 2010;35:436-8.
3. Sharma NC, Banavaliker JN, Ranjan R, et al. Bacteriological and epidemiological characteristics of diphtheria cases in and around Delhi—A retrospective study. Indian J Med Res. 2007;126:545-52.
4. WHO. (2018). Immunization, surveillance, assessment and monitoring. [online]. Available from http://www.who.int/entity/immunization_monitoring/data/incidence_series.xls [Accessed January, 2019].

CHAPTER 8

Otitis Media: Acute and Recurrent

Santanu Bhakta

Q1. What is otitis media?

A middle ear infection, also called *otitis media (OM)*, occurs when a virus or bacteria cause the area behind the eardrum to become inflamed. *OM is a middle ear infection that is most common in infants and young children, especially those between the ages of 6 months and 3 years.* By the age of 1 year, most children will have had one or more middle ear infections.

The term *OM* has two main categories: suppurative *acute otitis media (AOM)* and nonsuppurative *otitis media with effusion (OME)*. Middle ear effusion (MEE) signifies middle ear mucosal inflammation and a feature of both the conditions.

Q2. Which are the risk factors for AOM?

They include:

- Age between 6 months and 36 months old
- Using a pacifier
- Attending daycare
- Being bottle fed instead of breastfed (in infants)
- Drinking while laying down (in infants)
- Being exposed to cigarette smoke
- Being exposed to high levels of air pollution
- Experiencing changes in altitude
- Experiencing changes in climate
- Being in a cold climate
- Having had a recent cold, flu, sinus, or ear infection.

  Genetics also plays a role in increasing your child's risk of AOM.

Q3. What are MEE, OME, and AOM?

- Middle ear effusion should be considered, when we find either at least two of the following:
  - Limited mobility of tympanic membrane (TM)
  - Abnormal TM color

  - Opacification of TM not due to scarring
  - Air-fluid level behind TM
- Middle ear effusion without any acute inflammation is OME.
- Middle ear effusion with at least any one sign of acute inflammation (like, acute ear pain, marked redness of TM, and distinct bulging of the TM) is AOM.

Q4. What are the organisms responsible for AOM?

Both viral and bacterial pathogens are responsible. AOM occurs most frequently as a consequence of viral upper respiratory tract infection, causing eustachian tube dysfunction. The three most common bacterial pathogens in AOM are *Streptococcus pneumoniae,* nontypeable *Haemophilus influenzae,* and *Moraxella catarrhalis.* Other pathogens like *Staphylococcus aureus and gram-negative organisms* are commonly found in neonates.

Q5. How to diagnose AOM?

Otoscopy is a must for the diagnosis of AOM. According to 2013 American Academy of Pediatrics (AAP) guidelines, AOM should be diagnosed in children, who present with:

- Moderate to severe bulging of TM or new onset of otorrhea not due to acute otitis externa.
- Mild bulging of the TM and recent (less than 48 hours) onset of ear pain (holding, tugging, and rubbing of the ear in a nonverbal child) or intense erythema of the TM.
- Acute otitis media should not be diagnosed in children without MEE.

Q6. Why is it important to differentiate between AOM and OME?

In this era of limiting antibiotic use and preventing antimicrobial resistance, distinguishing OME from AOM is important in management, because OME in the absence of acute infection and does not require antibiotics.

Q7. What is the management for AOM?

The prime importance in managing AOM is assessment of pain. If pain is present, treatment should be started to reduce pain.

Q8. How should antibiotic therapy be initiated for treatment of AOM?

The fact that most cases of AOM resolve spontaneously, AAP consensus guidelines gives a breathing space between "initial observation" and "initial antibiotic therapy". A short period of watchful waiting for 24–48 hours rather than antibiotics may be appropriate for children over 6 months of age with minimal symptoms who do not have recurrent infections or structural differences in their ears, and are not at high risk for complications.

Initial observation is limited to symptomatic relief of pain and fever with commencement of antibiotic therapy only if the child's condition worsens at any time or does not improve within 48–72 hours of diagnosis.

Initial antibiotic therapy is when antibiotics are prescribed at the time of diagnosis. If the child has severe disease, especially below 2 years, prompt use of antibiotic is recommended.

Q9. During initial observation, how the child should be monitored?

In practicing initial observation with watchful waiting, age of the patient and laterality and severity of the disease should be considered carefully and the child should be assessed periodically for any worsening of symptoms.

Q10. When to start antibiotic therapy in children with AOM?

- In very young patients less than 6 months of age, even suspected cases of AOM should be treated with antibiotics because of increased chances of complications.
- Acute otitis media with otorrhea should always be treated with antibiotics at any age.
- Antibiotics should be started for bilateral or unilateral AOM in children 6 months and older with severe symptoms [i.e. moderate or severe otalgia or otalgia for at least 48 hours, or temperature 39°C (102.2°F) or higher].
- Antibiotics should be started for bilateral AOM in children younger than 24 months without severe signs or symptoms [i.e. mild otalgia for less than 48 hours and temperature less than 39°C (102.2°F)].
- Initial antibiotic therapy or initial observation with close follow-up for unilateral AOM in children 6–23 months of age without severe symptoms [i.e. mild otalgia for less than 48 hours and temperature less than 39°C (102.2°F)].
- In children 24 months or older with unilateral or bilateral AOM without severe signs or symptoms, either initial antibiotic therapy or initial observation with close follow-up should be offered.

Q11. Overview of AOM treatment options.

Child age	*Certain diagnosis*	*Uncertain diagnosis*
<6 months	Antibiotics	Antibiotics
6 months to 2 years	Antibiotics	Antibiotics if severe illness Observe if nonsevere illness
2 years and older	Antibiotics if severe illness	Observe if nonsevere illness

Antimicrobial therapy is significantly beneficial in younger children, children with otorrhea, and in bilateral AOM than in older children, without otorrhea or children with unilateral AOM.

Q12. How effective is antibiotic therapy for AOM?

Mainly three factors tilt the balance in favor of antibiotic therapy in documented cases of AOM:

- Fast symptomatic relief and resolution of infection
- Adequate prevention of suppurative complications
- A large proportion of cases are due to pathogenic bacteria.

Q13. What are the Centers for Disease Control and Prevention (CDC) guidelines for the use of antibiotics for treatment of acute AOM?

The CDC published six principles of appropriate antibiotic use in an attempt to reduce bacterial resistance. These principles are as follows:

1. Otitis media should be classified as AOM or OME
2. Antimicrobials are indicated for treatment of documented AOM only
3. Uncomplicated AOM in children older than 2 years may be treated with a course of antibiotics for 5–7 days
4. Antimicrobials are indicated for OME, if it persists for longer than 3 months
5. Persistent OME after full course of antimicrobial therapy for AOM does not require repeat antibiotics
6. Antimicrobial prophylaxis should be reserved for recurrent AOM, defined as three or more distinct and well-documented episodes in 6 months or four or more episodes in 12 months.

Q14. What is the basis of antibiotic selection in the treatment of AOM?

The antibiotic should cover most of the common etiological pathogens and must be individualized for the child with regard to allergy, tolerance, previous exposure to antibiotics, cost, and community resistance levels.

Q15. What is the first-line antibiotic of choice for AOM?

Amoxicillin (40 mg/kg/day) remains the drug of choice for uncomplicated AOM because of its high safety profile, excellent taste, easy availability, and low cost. It is very useful especially when a child has not received amoxicillin in the past 30 days or the child does not have concurrent purulent conjunctivitis (with ipsilateral OM signifies nontypeable *H. influenzae* infection; *otitis-conjunctivitis syndrome*) or the child is not allergic to penicillin. Increasing the dose from traditional 40–45 mg/kg/day to 80–90 mg/kg/day will provide efficacy against some penicillin-resistant strains. This higher dose should be used in children younger than 2 years and who received treatment with β-lactam drugs in past 30 days. High level penicillin resistance is not an issue for our country as of now.

Amoxicillin-clavulanate (40 mg/kg/day of amoxycillin with 6.4 mg/kg/day of clavulanate) is another first-line drug for AOM when the child has received amoxicillin in last 30 days or has concurrent purulent conjunctivitis, or has a history of recurrent AOM unresponsive to amoxicillin.

Q16. What is the alternative treatment in case of unsatisfactory response to first-line treatment?

Any second-line drugs should be effective against β-lactamase producing strains of nontypeable *H. influenza, M. catarrhalis*, and against nonsusceptible strains of *S. pneumoniae*. Only four drugs meet these criteria; cefdinir (14 mg/kg/day in two divided doses), cefuroxime (30 mg/kg/day in two divided doses), cefpodoxime (10 mg/kg/day in two divided doses), and ceftriaxone [50 mg/kg/day intramuscular (IM) or intravenous (IV) for 1–3 days] have been used with comparable efficacy.

Q17. What drugs are recommended in case of failure of initial antibiotic treatment for 48–72 hours?

Patient should always be reassessed for worsening of symptoms or failure in response to the initial antibiotic treatment within 48–72 hours and determine whether a change in therapy is needed. In that case, amoxicillin-clavulanate or ceftriaxone in recommended doses should be given. Other drugs that can be tried are clindamycin (30–40 mg/kg/day in three divided doses) with or without third-generation cephalosporin.

Q18. What about using macrolides or trimethoprim-sulfamethoxazole in treating AOM?

Many strains of nontypeable *H. influenzae* and *S. pneumoniae* are resistant to trimethoprim-sulfamethoxazole and also there is a high rate of clinical failure in children with this drug. Similarly, increasing rate of resistance against macrolides makes this drug unsuitable to treat AOM in children.

Q19. What is the duration of treatment?

Most efficacy studies have set the duration as 7–10 days. Longer duration is needed for a child less than 6 months with severe disease, child with craniofacial anomalies.

Q20. What is recurrent AOM and how is it managed?

When there are three episodes in 6 months or four episodes in 1 year duration with one episode in the preceding 6 months, it is called recurrent AOM. In that case, a second-line drug should be chosen to treat the case.

Q21. What is the role of antimicrobial prophylaxis?

It is better not to advice prophylactic antibiotics to reduce the frequency of episodes of AOM in children with recurrent AOM. In the past, it has been used in subtherapeutic doses, but now it is inadvisable due to the risk of increased antimicrobial resistance. A tympanostomy tube is another choice for recurrent AOM.

Q22. What is chronic suppurative otitis media (CSOM) and how it is managed?

Chronic suppurative otitis media is persistent middle ear infection with discharge through perforated TM. Most common etiologic agent is *Pseudomonas aeruginosa and S. aureus.* Rational approach should be microbiological culture and parenteral antibiotic.

Q23. Which are indications for tympanostomy tube insertion?

There is relatively strong evidence for tympanostomy tube insertion in children with chronic bilateral OME with associated significant hearing difficulties as well as in children with recurrent AOM with MEE. Tube insertion is optional, but recommended in children at risk for speech, language or learning problems who have recurrent AOM or OME, and in children who have chronic OME with symptoms. When making clinical decisions, the risks of tube insertion must be balanced against the risks of prolonged or recurrent OM, which include suppurative complications, damage to the TM, adverse effects of antibiotics, and potential developmental sequelae of hearing loss

Q24. What are the preventive measures and the role of vaccination in AOM?

Administration of pneumococcal conjugate vaccine to all children along with annual influenza vaccine is recommended according to the schedule.

Encourage exclusive breastfeeding for at least 6 months.

Encourage avoidance of tobacco smoke exposure [environmental tobacco smoke (ETS)].

FURTHER READING

1. Allan S. Lieberthal, Aaron E, et al. The diagnosis and management of acute otitis media. Pediatrics. 2013;131:e964-99.
2. Marcdante K, Kliegman R. Nelson Essentials of Pediatrics, 1st edition. Amsterdam, Netherlands: Elsevier; 2016.
3. NICE. (2018). Otitis media (acute): antimicrobial prescribing. [online] Available from https://www.nice.org.uk/guidance/ng91 [Accessed December 2018].

CHAPTER 9

Sinusitis

Ashok Rai

Q1. What is acute bacterial rhinosinusitis?

Sinusitis is defined as the inflammation of the paranasal sinuses and nasal cavity. Paranasal sinuses are an extension of upper respiratory tract and sinusitis is a usual complications of upper respiratory tract infections, almost always associated with rhinitis; hence rhinosinusitis is the preferred term. Uncomplicated viral sinusitis usually resolves in 7–10 days but if it continues beyond 10 days, possibility of secondary bacterial infection should be kept in mind. Numerous classification have been proposed for sinusitis.

Usually there are 4 conditions:

1. *Acute sinusitis:* Symptoms less than four weeks
2. *Subacute sinusitis*: Symptoms >4 weeks and <12 weeks
3. *Recurrent acute sinusitis*: Frequent multiple episodes per year with fewer complete resolution
4. *Chronic sinusitis*: Symptoms >12 weeks.

Q2. What are the predisposing factors for rhinosinusitis?

Viral upper respiratory infection and allergy are the most common predisposing factors for acute bacterial sinusitis. Other factors are; nasal polyps, foreign body, dental infections, cleft palate, ciliary dysfunction, cystic fibrosis and immunodeficiency.

Q3. What are usual clinical features of rhinosinusitis?

Usually these patients present with fever, cough, headache, facial pain, profuse mucopurulent discharge, and anosmia. Young infants and children may present with irritability. As per European position paper on rhinosinusitis 2012, the presence of two or more symptoms, one of which should be either nasal blockage/obstruction/congestion or nasal discharge for a minimum of 3 days, associated with facial pain, cough, fever, malaise and/either endoscopic signs of mucopurulent discharge and/or computed tomography (CT) changes are helpful in diagnosing rhinosinusitis.

Q4. What are the causative organisms for acute bacterial rhinosinusitis?

Causative organisms for the sinusitis are usually viral, mainly rhinoviruses, adenoviruses or parainfluenza. The common bacterial organisms are *Streptococcus pneumoniae,* nontypeable *Haemophilus influenzae, Moraxella catarrhalis* and *Streptococcus pyogenes.*

Chronic sinusitis is usually a polymicrobial infection. The usual pathogens for chronic sinusitis are alpha hemolytic streptococci, *Staphylococcus aureus,* coagulase negative staphylococci, nontypeable *H. influenzae, Moraxella catarrhalis,* anerobic bacteria, bacteroides, etc.

Q5. How will you diagnose sinusitis?

Diagnosis of bacterial sinusitis is mainly clinical. Radiographic studies and other modalities like CT scanning, confirms the sinus inflammation but cannot differentiate the causes of sinusitis. As per the American Academy of Pediatrics guidelines, laboratory diagnosis is required in only a few patients, who do not recover or worsen during the course of antimicrobial treatment.

The main challenge is to differentiate viral upper respiratory illness (URI) from bacterial sinus infection. Purulent secretions in the middle meatus are highly suggestive of bacterial infection.

Computed tomography/magnetic resonance imaging (CT/MRI) is indicated in patients who have symptoms or signs of complicated sinusitis, such as focal neurologic deficits, periorbital edema or severe headache.

Q6. How will you manage sinusitis?

Main focus in treatment of rhinosinusitis are to reduce tissue edema, facilitate drainage and infection control. Since *Streptococcus pneumoniae, Haemophilus influenzae and Moraxella catarrhalis* are the common etiologic agents, we should choose antibiotics which cover all three organisms. The severity of clinical illness, recent exposure to antibiotics and other factors that increase the likelihood of infection with resistant bacterial pathogens should always be considered before starting the antibiotics.

First-line of therapy in bacterial sinusitis is Amoxicillin because of its effectiveness, safety, low cost and narrow spectrum. This should be used in dosages of 45 mg/kg/day in 2–3 divided dosages. However, high dose amoxicillin (90 mg/kg/day in 2 divided dosages) is indicated for penicillin resistant *Streptococcus pneumoniae* infection and in immunocompromised individuals. Drug resistance to *S. pneumoniae* is still low in India. Children attending day care centers, and those with a history of recent therapy with penicillin group, are at a risk of developing resistant infections and high dose amoxicillin may be advised.

Second-line treatment is indicated, when there is no clinical response after 48–72 hours of initiating therapy, or there is high incidence of beta lactamase producing organisms in the community. Amoxicillin-Clavulanate 45 mg/kg/day should be used to cover beta lactamase producing organisms.

For patient who are allergic to penicillin

- *Cefdinir*:14 mg/kg/day in two divided doses
- *Cefpodoxime*: 10 mg/kg/day in two divided doses
- *Cefuroxime*: 30 mg/kg/day in 2 divided dosages.

For severe beta lactam allergy

- *Clarithromycin*: 15 mg/kg/day in 2 divided dose
- *Azithromycin*: 10 mg/kg/day
- *Clindamycin*: 30–40 mg/kg/day in 4 divided dose.

Azithromycin is no longer recommended for the treatment of sinusitis, owing to high rates of resistance among both *S. pneumoniae and H. influenzae* isolates.

Q7. How long treatment should be given in sinusitis?

The American Academy of Pediatrics recommends minimum 10 days course of antibiotics in children. So, the usual duration of antibiotic therapy is 10–14 days or for 7 days beyond the resolution of symptoms, whichever is later.

Q8. What are the antimicrobial resistance pattern in organisms causing upper respiratory tract infection (URTI)?

S. pneumoniae develops resistance to penicillin by developing efflux mechanisms and by altering the penicillin binding proteins. Though, penicillin resistant *S. pneumoniae* are common in western countries, their incidence is still low in India.

H. influenzae and M. catarrhalis produce beta lactamases, which directly degrades beta lactam ring of amino penicillin. Beta lactam resistance is mediated either by production of enzymes capable of hydrolyzing beta lactam ring or alteration of penicillin binding proteins. Majority of *Moraxella isolate* (95%) & some of *H. influenzae* (25–30%) are beta lactamase producing and resistant to penicillin. They can be treated with Amoxicillin-Clavulanate combinations.

Q9. Are there any role of adjuvant therapies in sinusitis?

Adjuvant therapies include saline nasal irrigation, antihistamine, decongestants, topical intra nasal steroids and mucolytic agents. Available evidences do not recommend the use of adjuvant therapies. There is no role of antimicrobial prophylaxis in children with recurrent episodes of acute bacterial sinusitis.

FURTHER READING

1. Chen CF, Wu KG, Hsu MC, et al. Prevalence and relationship between allergic diseases and infectious diseases. J Microbiol Immunol Infect. 2001;34:57-62.
2. Chow AW, Benniger MS, Brook I, et al. IDSA clinical practice guidelines for acute bacterial rhinosinusitis in children and adults. Clin Infect Dis. 2012;54:72-112.
3. Fokkens WJ, Lund VJ, Mullol J, et al. European position paper on rhinosinusitis and nasal polyps 2012. Rhinol. 2012;23:1-298.
4. Malaty J. Medical management of chronic rhinosinusitis in adults. Sinusitis. 2016;1:76-88.
5. Parthasarthy A, Kundu R, Yewale V, et al. Textbook of Pediatric Infectious Diseases. 2nd edition Jaypee Brothers Medical Publishers. New Delhi;2019. pp. 160-2.
6. Runkle K. Decongestants, antihistamines and nasal irrigation for acute sinusitis in children. Paediatr Child Health. 2016;2(3):143-4.
7. Singhal T, Shah N. Rational anti-microbial practice in pediatrics. 2nd edition. Jaypee Brother Medical Publishers, New Delhi; 2014. pp. 203-4.
8. Wald ER, Applegate KE, Bordley C, et al. Clinical practice guidelines for the diagnosis and management of acute bacterial sinusitis in children aged 1 to 18 years. American Academy of Pediatrics (AAP). Pediatrics. 2013;132:1-21.

CHAPTER 10

Whooping Cough

Parang N Mehta

Q1. What causes whooping cough/pertussis?

Pertussis, also known as whooping cough, is a highly contagious respiratory disease. It is caused by the bacterium *Bordetella pertussis,* a gram-negative coccobacillus. A small percentage of cases are caused by *Bordetella parapertussis,* which causes a similar but less protracted illness.

Pertussis is a disease characterized by severe, spasmodic cough, and a protracted course.

Pertussis is known for uncontrollable, violent coughing which often makes it hard to breathe. After coughing bouts, someone with pertussis often needs to take deep breaths, which result in a "whooping" sound. Pertussis can affect people of all ages, but can be very serious, even deadly for babies less than a year old.

Similar pertussoid cough can also be caused by mycoplasma species, adenoviruses, parainfluenza or influenza viruses, enteroviruses, and respiratory syncytial virus.

Q2. Are antibiotics needed for whooping cough?

The medical management of pertussis cases is primarily supportive, although antibiotics are of some value. This therapy eradicates the organism from secretions, thereby decreasing communicability and, if initiated early, may modify the course of the illness. The basic goals of management are to assess the progression of the disease, the likelihood of life-threatening events, and to prevent or treat complications. Good supportive care towards nutrition, rest, and recovery without sequelae is the cornerstone of pertussis management.

Q3. What are the aims of antibiotic therapy?

There are two aims:

1. Antibiotics, if started in the catarrhal stage, shorten the course of the disease and reduce complications. However, it is difficult to diagnose pertussis at this stage.

2. The second aim of antibiotic therapy in a child with pertussis is reduced infectivity. Pertussis is highly infectious, and people around a case are at high risk. A course of antibiotics renders the child noninfectious. The child should be isolated for 5 days after antibiotics are begun.

Q4. Which antibiotics are recommended for pertussis?

Bordetella pertussis is susceptible to the macrolides, quinolones, third-generation cephalosporins, and meropenem. First- and second-generation cephalosporins are not effective, and ampicillin is moderately effective.

The drug of choice is the macrolides.

- *Azithromycin-dose*:
  - Infants aged less than 6 months: 10 mg/kg per day for 5 days.
  - Infants and children aged more than or equal to 6 months: 10 mg/kg (maximum: 500 mg) on day 1, followed by 5 mg/kg per day (maximum: 250 mg) on days 2–5.
- Erythromycin (40–50 mg/kg/day in four divided doses for 14 days) and azithromycin are commonly used, and resistance rates are low in most parts of the world.
- Clarithromycin can also be used (15–20 mg/kg/day in two divided doses for 7–10 days).

They are most effective if started in the catarrhal stage, at which time diagnosis is rarely made. Starting antibiotics in the paroxysmal stage has lesser clinical benefit, but reduces infectivity. Erythromycin should be avoided in neonates, because of an association with infantile hypertrophic pyloric stenosis. For infants aged less than 1 month, azithromycin is preferred; erythromycin and clarithromycin are not recommended.

Q5. Are antibiotics needed for prophylaxis?

Pertussis is one of the most infectious diseases known. Secondary attack rates are close to 100% among close contacts. An antibiotic effective against pertussis should be administered to all close contacts of persons with pertussis, regardless of age and vaccination status.

Administration of postexposure prophylaxis to asymptomatic household contacts within 21 days of onset of cough in the index patient can prevent symptomatic infection. Coughing (symptomatic) household members of a pertussis patient should be treated as if they have pertussis. Because severe and sometimes fatal pertussis-related complications occur in infants aged less than 12 months, especially among infants aged less than 4 months, postexposure prophylaxis should be administered in exposure settings that include infants aged less than 12 months or women in the third trimester of pregnancy. All contacts of the patient should be started on erythromycin

(40–50 mg/kg/day in four divided doses for 14 days) and azithromycin (10 mg/kg/day for 5 days) as soon as possible. Prophylaxis must be given even to fully immunized contacts.

FURTHER READING

1. CDC. (2005). Recommended Antimicrobial Agents for the Treatment and Postexposure Prophylaxis of Pertussis: 2005 CDC Guidelines. [online] Available from https://www.cdc.gov/mmwr/preview/mmwrhtml/rr5414a1.htm [Accessed December 2018].

CHAPTER 11

Community-acquired Pneumonias

Sanjay K Ghorpade

Q1. What is the etiology of community-acquired pneumonia (CAP)?

Age is the most important criteria to predict etiological agent for starting empiric treatment.

0–3 months: Gram-negative, *Chlamydia trachomatis*, viruses, and *Streptococcus pneumoniae.*

3–60 months age: Viruses (35%), bacteria (60%) which includes *Haemophilus influenzae, S. pneumoniae*, staphylococci, *Mycoplasma* (24–30%) more in above 5 years, chlamydia (6–11%), and mixed infections (9%).

Q2. What are clues to etiology?

Predisposing factors	*Organism*
• Pyoderma and measles	*Staphylococcus*
• Human immunodeficiency virus (HIV)	*Pneumocystis*
• Neutropenia	Gram-negative and *Aspergillus*
• Cystic fibrosis	*Pseudomonas* and *Staphylococcus*
• Severe protein-energy malnutrition (PEM)	Gram-negative and *Staphylococcus*
• Aspiration pneumonia	Anaerobes

Clinical/laboratory clues to etiology:

- Outbreak setting: *Mycoplasma* and viral
- Young febrile infant with neonatal conjunctivitis: Chlamydia
- Multisystem involvement with hepatitis, rash, and anemia: *Mycoplasma*
- Low white blood cell (WBC), low platelet count, high creatine phosphokinase (CPK), and high serum glutamic-oxaloacetic transaminase (SGOT): Influenza
- Pneumatocele on X-ray: Staphylococcal
- Persistent pneumonia with significant lymphadenopathy, military shadow, fibrocavitary lesions: Tuberculosis (TB).

Q3. How will you diagnose pneumonia?

Diagnosis is always clinical. It should be suspected in any child having fever and rapid breathing with or without cough. Fever, tachypnea, nasal flaring (in infants), and reduced oxygen saturation are predictive of pneumonia. These findings, especially in infants, are highly specific and greatly increase the likelihood of pneumonia when present. However, their absence does not rule out pneumonia, and the accuracy of any individual sign or symptom is limited. In addition to fever and tachypnea there will be decreased breath sounds, crackles, dull percussion note, and bronchial breathing in the affected area.

Q4. Which tests are available to determine etiology of pneumonia?

Complete blood count (CBC) and C-reactive protein (CRP) are nonspecific and will provide evidence of infection only.

- Some times X-ray chest may give important clue, e.g. pneumatocele on X-ray in staphylococcal and persistent pneumonia with significant lymphadenopathy, milliary shadow, fibrocavitary lesions, etc. in a case of TB.

For microbial diagnosis blood cultures, sputum/BAL Gram stain and culture, pleural fluid Gram stain and culture, serologic tests for *Mycoplasma* and chlamydia, and *Pneumococcus* (antigen detection in urine and pleural fluid), and molecular tests for viruses are carried out.

Q5. Are these tests really required?

They are not needed in a simple CAP in an immunocompetent child. They are rarely indicated for nonresponding, persistent, and recurrent pneumonia.

Limitations:

- *Culture from respiratory tract*: Sputum sample collection is difficult and invasive methods such as bronchoalveolar lavage (BAL) and lung puncture not justified routinely. Pleural fluid cultures also have poor yield.
- *Blood culture*: Yield is poor [blood culture and sensitivity (C/S) positivity 15%].
- *Serologic tests*: Available only for *Mycoplasma*; poor sensitivity/specificity, expensive and available as a panel.
- *Molecular diagnosis*: Expensive and not easily available.
- Not recommended at all for outpatients. May be done for inpatients.
- Indicated for immunocompromised, nonresponding and nosocomial pneumonias, and children with comorbidities.

Q6. How to choose empiric antibiotics for CAP (outpatient)?

Age	*First-line*	*Second-line*
3 months to 5 years	Amoxicillin*	Co-amoxiclav/cefuroxime
>5 years	Amoxicillin*	Macrolide**/Co-amoxiclav/cefuroxime

Note: Less than 3 months treat as inpatients.
*Standard doses 30–50 mg/kg/day
**Erythromycin/clarithromycin/azithromycin

Q7. How to choose empiric antibiotics for CAP (inpatients)?

Age	*Antibiotic choice*
<3 months	Cefotaxime/ceftriaxone ± aminoglycoside
3 months to 5 years	Co-amoxiclav/ceftriaxone/cefotaxime
>5 years	Ampicillin/penicillin G/co-amoxiclav/ceftriaxone/cefotaxime and macrolides (if *Mycoplasma* is suspected)
Suspected *Staphylococcus*	Cefuroxime Or co-amoxiclav Or IV third-generation cephalosporins + cloxacillin [vancomycin/teicoplanin/linezolid, if methicillin-resistant *Staphylococcus aureus* (MRSA) is suspected]

As the incidence of drug-resistant *Streptococcus pneumoniae* (DRSP) is currently low in India, standard doses of amoxicillin are usually adequate. Erythromycin/azithromycin/clarithromycin are equally efficacious but differ in terms of side effects, cost, drug interactions, duration of therapy, and acceptability. Azithromycin is probably the preferred drug on these counts.

Q8. What could be reasons for nonresponse to amoxicillin in 3 months to 5 years?

- *Resistance*: Beta-lactamase producing *H. influenzae* and hence switch to co-amoxiclav is recommended. Chloramphenicol though cheaper, is more toxic and about 40% of *H. influenzae* is resistant to both amoxicillin/chloramphenicol.
- Drug-resistant *S. pneumoniae* especially high level resistance.
- *Alternative etiology*: Viral pneumonia/*Mycoplasma*.
- Complications such as empyema, thrombophlebitis, drug fever, and underlying foreign body.

Q9. What could be reasons for nonresponse to amoxicillin in more than 5 years?

- Alternative etiology such as *Mycoplasma* and hence addition/switch to a macrolide is recommended.
- Drug-resistant *S. pneumoniae* especially high level resistance.

- The likelihood of *H. influenzae* is low at this age.
- Complications as mentioned above.

Cefotaxime and ceftriaxone are preferred agents for inpatient management of CAP if resources permit because they cover resistant *H. influenzae* and all DRSP. Aminoglycosides are particularly indicated in neonates.

Vancomycin is inferior to cloxacillin in methicillin-sensitive *S. aureus* (MSSA). Vancomycin is currently considered inferior to linezolid for management of suspected methicillin-resistant *S. aureus* (MRSA) pneumonia due to poor penetration in lung tissue.

Q10. What is the need for empirical anti-influenza drug in CAP?

Radical change in treatment after the novel H1N1 epidemic.

During a notified outbreak, all patients who meet the definition of pneumonia should also be given oseltamivir in addition to antibiotics. Not possible to differentiate viral from bacterial pneumonia clinically/lab. Definitive treatment of influenza pneumonia is with the neuraminidase inhibitor drugs oseltamivir and zanamivir. Oseltamivir is the first-line drug and zanamivir should be used in those with oseltamivir resistant virus. These drugs reduce duration of symptoms, risk of complications and death. Though they are most effective if given within the first 48 hours of illness; but are useful even if given later at any time point of a severe illness.

The therapeutic dose of oseltamivir is 30 mg twice daily in those with weight less than 15 kg, 45 mg twice daily for 15–24 kg, 60 mg twice daily for 25–34 kg and 75 mg twice daily for those 35 kg and above. Oseltamivir though formally not approved for infants, is generally safe and may be used in a dose of 2–3 mg/kg twice daily. The duration of therapy is 5 days. In patients with very severe disease double the recommended dose for 10 days may be used. Oseltamivir is well tolerated with occasional gastrointestinal (GI) and neurological side effects.

The novel H1N1 virus is resistant to amantadine.

Q11. What are common causes of nonresolution even after appropriate antibiotics therapy?

- *Complications*: Empyema and lung abscess
- *Bacterial resistance*: MRSA, ESBL, *Klebsiella*, DRSP, etc.
- *Other Bugs*: *Mycoplasma* and TB
- Nonbacterial etiology
- *Bronchial obstruction*: Foreign body (FB), gland, tumor
- Pre-existing diseases
- Noninfectious causes
- Immunocompromised host.

Q12. When will you suspect staphylococcal pneumonia?

- In young children with CAP:
  - Severely ill, have current or recent influenza, whose symptoms do not improve with beta-lactam or macrolide antibiotic therapy.
- In older children:
  - Signs of pneumonia with proceeding skin lesions like abscess, or furuncles as in the first case. History of measles in a recent past is also a risk factor.

Q13. What are radiologic findings of *S. aureus* pneumonia?

- Although not specific to *S. aureus* the following signs are very suggestive of a staphylococcal disease:
  - Pneumatoceles, empyema/loculated fluid, air leaks, pneumothorax, hydropneumothorax, pneumopericardium, and bilateral fluffy infiltrates.

Q14. What are antibiotics for staphylococcal pneumonia?

- Methicillin-sensitive *S. aureus:*
  - Cloxacillin the best
  - Cefazolin equally good alternative
  - Ceftriaxone—effective but inferior to cloxacillin or cefazolin
  - Clindamycin effective (antitoxin effect)
  - Vancomycin and linezolid inferior to beta-lactams
- Methicillin-resistant *S. aureus:*
  - Vancomycin best suited for bacteremia
  - Clindamycin effective alternative for pneumonia alone
  - Linezolid—oral switch feasible
  - Daptomycin ineffective.

Q15. When to do follow-up X-ray?

Repeat X-ray is indicated in a nonresponding child with clinical deterioration or no clinical improvement after 3–4 days of appropriate antibiotic. In a clinically improving child X-ray may take 2–3 weeks for complete resolution.

It may be required in a nonresolving, recurrent pneumonia, or when alternative diagnosis is to be confirmed or ruled out.

Q16. How do you diagnose atypical pneumonia?

More commonly seen in a child after 5 years of age. The usual presentation seems to be like viral illness with malaise, headache, sore throat, ear infections, lower fevers (101–102), usually nonproductive, and persistent cough. Usually it involves interstitial lung tissue and may or may not have rales. The subjective symptoms are out of proportion to lung involvement.

Q17. What are the indications for macrolides in pneumonia?

- Clues to atypical pneumonia present clinically or radiologically
- Extrapulmonary manifestations
- No response to first-line antibiotics
- Pertussis with CAP.

Q18. What about macrolide-resistant *Mycoplasma*?

Fluoroquinolones can be used for atypical pneumonia not responding to macrolides.

Q19. What is the appropriate antibiotic therapy for aspiration pneumonia?

- Community-acquired aspiration pneumonia is usually treated with amoxicillin-clavulanate.
- Clindamycin is an alternative for patients allergic to penicillin.

Q20. How to prevent CAP?

- Exclusive breastfeeding (BF) up to first 6 months
- Good nutrition
- Protect from passive smoking
- Vitamin D, zinc, and vitamin A supplements
- *Vaccine*: Bacillus Calmette–Guérin (BCG), diphtheria, tetanus, pertussis/ diphtheria, tetanus, acellular pertussis (DTP/DTaP), *Haemophilus influenzae* type b (Hib), influenza, pneumococcal vaccines, measles containing vaccine, and chickenpox vaccine.

FURTHER READING

1. Feldman C, Anderson R. Controversies in the treatment of pneumococcal community-acquired pneumonia. Future Microbiol. 2006;1(3):271-81.
2. Fuller JD, Low DE. A review of *Streptococcus pneumoniae* infection treatment failures associated with fluoroquinolone resistance. Clin Infect Dis. 2005;41(1):118-21.
3. Kim SH, Song JH, Chung DR, et al. Changing trend of antimicrobial resistance and serotypes in Streptococcus pneumoniae in Asian countries: an ANSORP study. Antimicrob Agents Chemother. 2012;56(3):1418-26.
4. Kliegman RM, St Geme J, Schor NF (Eds). Nelson Text Book of Pediatrics, 20th edition. Philadelphia: Elsevier; 2016.
5. McIntosh K. Community-acquired pneumonia in children. N Engl J Med. 2002;346(6):429-37.
6. Nguyen TKP, Tran TH, Robert CL, et al. Child pneumonia in the Western Pacific Region. Paediatr Respir Rev. 2017;21:102-10.
7. Parthasarathy A. Textbook of Pediatric Infectious Diseases, 2nd edition. New Delhi: Jaypee Brothers Medical Publishers (P) Ltd.; 2003.

8. Peterson LR. Penicillins for treatment of pneumococcal pneumonia: does in vitro resistance really matter? Clin Infect Dis. 2006;42(2):224-33.
9. WHO. (2016). World Health Statistics 2016: Monitoring health for the SDGs. [online] Available from http://www.who.int/gho/publications/world_health_statistics/2016/en/ [Accessed January, 2019].
10. Yoshida LM, Suzuki M, Thiem VD, et al. Population based cohort study for pediatric infectious diseases research in Vietnam. Trop Med Health. 2014;42(2):S47-58.

CHAPTER 12

Empyema

Kheya Ghosh Uttam

Q1. What is empyema?

Empyema is presence of pus or microorganism in the pleural fluid. Most cases of empyema develop as a complication of pneumonia. The disease can also be produced by rupture of a lung abscess into the pleural space, by contamination introduced from trauma or thoracic surgery, rarely, by mediastinitis or the extension of intra-abdominal abscesses.

Q2. What are the common organisms responsible for empyema?

Empyema is commonly associated with pneumonia due to *Streptococcus pneumonia, Streptococcus pyogenes* and *Staphylococcus aureus. Staphylococcus aureus* is the most common in developing countries and in post-traumatic empyema. Since the introduction of Hib vaccine the relative incidence of *Haemophilus influenzae* empyema has decreased. Group A *Streptococcus, Klebsiella aerogenes, Escherichia coli,* tuberculosis, fungi, and parasites are less common causes. Anaerobes and enterobacter are common in mixed infection. For anaerobes, aspiration pneumonia is the most common cause followed by lung abscess, subdiaphragmatic abscess and spreading infection from adjacent sites. *Aspergillus fumigatus* and *Candida albicans* are fungi which can cause empyema, especially in immunocompromised children. *Entamoeba histolytica* may cause empyema if a subdiaphragmatic abscess burst in pleural cavity.

Q3. How to decide on the antibiotic therapy of empyema?

All children with empyema will need antibiotic therapy. It is important to ensure pleural penetration for effective therapy so intravenous high doses in the early stages of the disease are recommended. As the most common organisms responsible for empyema are *Streptococcus pneumoniae, Streptococcus pyogenes, Staphylococcus aureus,* it is recommended that the initial empirical choice of antibiotics should cover at least *Streptococcus pneumoniae* and *Staphylococcus aureus.* Intravenous cloxacillin along with injection 3rd generation cephalosporin is used as initial therapy.

Other alternatives include co-amoxiclav. Aminoglycosides can be added in suspected *S. aureus* case for its synergistic action. Monotherapy with aminoglycosides is contraindicated as they have poor activity in the pus.

Community-acquired MRSA infection is on rise and so clindamycin is often added for the treatment of complicated community-acquired pneumonia. Intravenous vancomycin is the drug of choice for MRSA. *S. pneumoniae* with high level of resistance to penicillin and 3rd generation cephalosporins should be treated with vancomycin.

Anaerobic infection should be considered in those children at risk of aspiration and so metronidazole or clindamycin should be added.

There is no need to routinely use a macrolide antibiotic but its use should be considered in *Mycoplasma pneumoniae* infection. However, *Mycoplasma pneumoniae* vary rarely causes empyema in children, particularly in the under 5-year-old population.

Broader spectrum coverage like meropenem is often required for hospital-acquired infection as well as those secondary to surgery, trauma and aspirations.

Q4. What should be the duration of antibiotic treatment?

Antibiotic should be continued until the patient is afebrile , total leucocyte count normalizes, thoracostomy tube drains less than 50 mL of fluid per day and chest X-ray shows considerable clearing. Normally *H. influenzae* and *S. pneumoniae* needs 7–14 days course of antibiotics while *S. aureus* need 3–4 weeks. Duration of therapy for anaerobic empyema is variable depending on whether lung lesions go on to cavitate. Often 6–12 weeks are required before the lung lesions get cleared or a small residual lesion is left.

Q5. What are the other associated treatments essential for empyema?

- *Empyema drainage*: Chest tube drainage is an essential component of empyema treatment. A chest tube with an underwater seal should be placed. The chest tube must be kept inside till drainage is less than 30–50 mL/day.
- *Thrombolytic therapy*: Useful in multiloculated empyema. Streptokinase and urokinase are used as thrombolytics.
- *Surgical modalities*: Video-assisted thoracoscopic surgical (VATS), thoracoscopic debridement and irrigation and decortication.

Q6. What is the role of fibrinolytic agents in the management of pediatric empyema?

Benefit of use of fibrinolytics in empyema is inconsistent across various studies. Evidence is still not sufficient to recommend routine use. Intrapleural fibrinolytics are recommended for any complicated parapneumonic effusion (thick fluid with loculations). Three types of fibrinolytics are available in clinical use namely streptokinase, urokinase and alteplase out of which urokinase is not available in India. Several case series in children using these agents reported successful outcome without surgery in 90%. Few trial also showed the length of hospital stay in fibrinolytic treated group was significantly low (specially in favor of urokinase) whereas few recent studies failed to show any benefit. At present there is no evidence to suggest which of the three fibrinolytic agents is most effective, but only urokinase has been studied in a randomized controlled trial in children and so it is recommended. As urokinase is not available in India and alteplase is quite expensive, streptokinase is often used in our country.

Q7. What is the role of VATS?

Video-assisted thoracoscopic surgery has its most appropriate role in early surgery as the failure rate is higher in advanced organized empyema, which often needs open thoracotomy and drainage later. The advantages are it is safe, has less postoperative pain, shorter hospital stay and a better cosmetic results. Contraindications for VATS include an inability to develop a pleural window to access the pleural cavity, the presence of thick pyogenic material and/or fibrotic pleural rinds.

CHAPTER 13

Suppurative Lung Diseases

Kheya Ghosh Uttam

Q1. What are the different suppurative lung conditions found in children?
The most frequent clinical suppurative lung conditions in children are empyema, lung abscess and bronchiectasis and less frequent condition is necrotizing pneumonia. A chronic neutrophil dominated bronchitis also known as persistent bacterial bronchitis (PBB) is also described.

Q2. What is lung abscess?
Lung abscess developed due to infection that leads to destruction of parenchyma, cavitation, and central necrosis. Lung abscesses are much less common in children than in adults. Lung abscesses may be primary or secondary. If lung abscess develops in a previously healthy patient with no underlying medical disorders it is known as primary lung abscess. A secondary abscess occurs in a patient with underlying or predisposing conditions.

Q3. Which organisms cause lung abscess?
Lung abscess is mainly polymicrobial. Both anaerobic and aerobic organisms can cause lung abscesses. Rarely parasitic and fungal infection causes lung abscess especially in immunocompromised children. Common anaerobic bacteria that can cause pulmonary abscess are found in oral cavity and include *Bacteroides, Fusobacterium,* and *Peptostreptococcus.* Abscesses can be caused by aerobic organisms such as *Streptococcus pneumoniae, Streptococcus pyogenes, Staphylococcus aureus, Escherichia coli, Klebsiella pneumoniae,* and *Pseudomonas aeruginosa, H. influenzae, actinomyces, nocardia and mycobacteria.* All patients with lung abscess should have aerobic and anaerobic cultures as part of their work-up. Fungi can also cause lung abscesses, particularly in immunocompromised patients. The common fungi are *Aspergillus, Cryptococcus, Histoplasma* and *Candida* species.

Q4. What are the different modes of management of lung abscess in children?
Management is mainly conservative treatment with antibiotics. A 2–3 weeks course of parenteral antibiotics for uncomplicated cases, followed by a course of oral antibiotics to complete a total of 4–6 weeks is recommended.

Choice of antibiotic should be guided by microbiological report of Gram stain and culture but initially should cover both aerobic and anaerobic organisms. Treatment regimens should include a penicillinase-resistant agent active against *S. aureus* and anaerobic coverage, typically with clindamycin.

Clindamycin is preferred over metronidazole as it has a good intracellular penetration and is stable in low pH.

Recommended combination of antibiotics for lung abscess is clindamycin along with a beta lactam-beta lactamase inhibitors, chloramphenicol, second generation cephalosporins, newer generation fluoroquinolones or meropenem. Aminoglycoside should not be used since they poorly pass through fibrous pyogenic membrane of chronic abscess.

Vancomycin or linezolid is recommended in lung abscess due to MRSA.

Surgical intervention should be considered in severely ill patients or those who fail to improve after 7–10 days of appropriate antimicrobial therapy. Minimally invasive percutaneous aspiration techniques, often with computed tomography (CT) guidance, are the initial and, often, only intervention. In rare complicated cases, thoracotomy with lobectomy and/or decortication may be necessary.

BRONCHIECTASIS

Q5. What are the predisposing factors for development of bronchiectasis in children?

Cystic fibrosis is the most common cause of bronchiectasis in children. Other conditions associated with bronchiectasis are combined under the heading of noncystic fibrosis bronchiectasis and include airway clearance abnormality such as ciliary dyskinesia, airway obstruction or anomalies such as airway malacia, extrinsic compression of airway, immune deficiency syndromes (Primary and acquired immunodeficiencies), and infection, especially pertussis, measles, adenovirus and tuberculosis.

Q6. What are the common organisms found in the bronchiectatic airways?

In bronchiectasis, the thickening and dilatation of the distal bronchi and bronchioles leads to retention of mucus and impaired clearance of the secretion which helps in bacterial proliferation. A wide variety of pathogenic bacteria such as *Staphylococcus, Streptococcus, Pneumococcus, H. influenzae,* anaerobes, *Pseudomonas* and microaerophilic bacteria can be found in the bronchiectatic airways.

Q7. What antimicrobial therapy is used in case of exacerbation of pulmonary infections in noncystic fibrosis bronchiectasis?

Antimicrobial therapy is based on the pattern of airway colonization for each patient. Empirically, treatment should be started with co-amoxiclav or with second or third generation cephalosporins to cover most common pathogens present in the bronchiectatic airway. Recommended treatments according to the organisms are given in **Table 1**. Antimicrobial therapy should be continued for at least 10–14 days. If oral therapy fails or the child is seriously ill, intravenous antibiotic is recommended.

Table 1: Recommended antimicrobial treatment for the common organism causing acute exacerbation of bronchiectasis.*

Microorganism	*First-line antibiotic*	*Second-line antibiotic*
S. pneumoniae	Amoxicillin	Macrolide
H. influenzae (beta lactam negative)	Amoxicillin	Macrolide or ceftriaxone
H. influenzae (Beta lactam positive)	Co-amoxiclav	Macrolide or ceftriaxone (IV)
Moraxella catarrhalis	Co-amoxiclav	Ciprofloxacin
MSSA	Trimethoprim/ sulfamethoxazole	Macrolide
MRSA—oral	Trimethoprim/ sulfamethoxazole	Rifampicin +doxycycline Third-line: Linezolid
MRSA-intravenous	Vancomycin	Linezolid
Klebsiella, Enterobacter spp.	Ciprofloxacin	IV Ceftriaxone
Pseudomonas aeruginosa	Ciprofloxacin	*Monotherapy*: IV ceftazidime or piperacillin tazobactam or aztreonam or meropenem *Polytherapy*: The above combined with either tobramycin or gentamicin or colistin

*British Thoracic Society guidelines for non-CF-Bronchiectasis.

CHAPTER 14

Acute Diarrheal Disorders

Chetan Shah

Q1. What are the indications of use of antibiotics in diarrhea?

Although majority of acute watery diarrhea patients do not need antibiotics. There are some indications for prescription for patients.

The most common indications are:

- Visible blood and in stool
- Diarrhea associated with systemic infections like pneumonia, otitis media (parenteral diarrhea)
- Diarrhea in immunocompromised host like in severe acute malnutrition (SAM) or human immunodeficiency virus (HIV) positive child or on child receiving chemotherapy
- Proven case of amebiasis, giardiasis or cholera
- Diarrhea in very young less than 3-month-old infant
- Pseudomembranous colitis
- Traveler's diarrhea
- Prolonged diarrhea
- Antibiotic-associated diarrhea (*Clostridium difficile*).

Q2. What are the criteria for use of antibiotics?

Use of antibiotics is described in **Flowchart 1**.

Q3. If stool examination shows pus cells, should you give antibiotics?

Mere presence of pus cells does not warrant antibiotics treatment. Presence of sheets of pus cells is an indication of bacterial infection. Routine stool examination and cultures have very poor specificity for diagnosing bacterial infections.

Q4. What are the common antibiotics suggested? Many taskforce including Indian Academy of Pediatrics (IAP) suggest co-trimoxazole as first-line drug, but often we do not get desired response with co-trimoxazole use. What should be the first-line antibiotic?

Flowchart 1: Schematic diagram for antibiotic use.

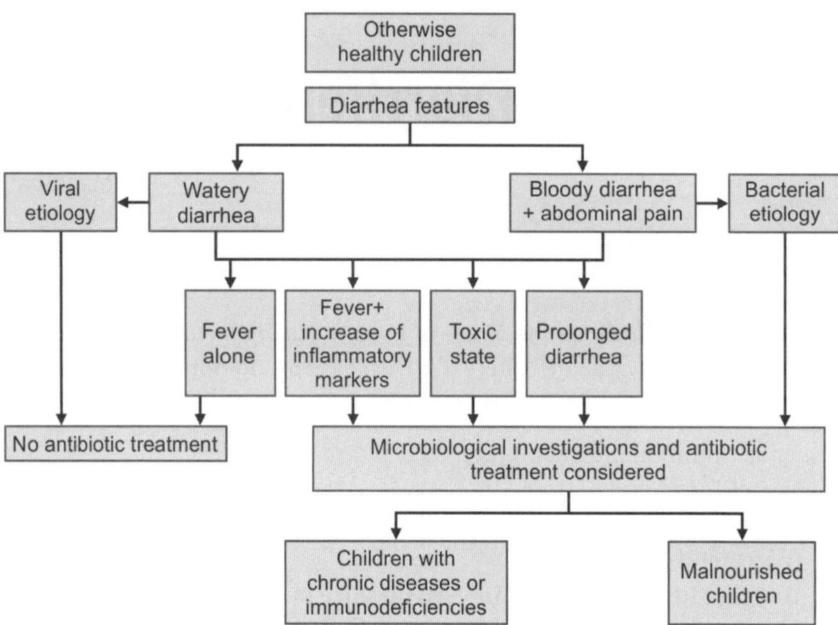

Unfortunately in India, we do not have robust microbiological data and lot of more studies are required to publish antibiotic recommendation for the entire country.

Antibiotics suggested are:
- Third-generation cephalosporins like cefixime and ceftriaxone
- Quinolones—nalidixic acid and ciprofloxacin
- Doxycycline—cholera
- Macrolides—campylobacter jejuni.

Q5. Various combinations are available containing antibiotic + metronidazole, ornidazole, and nitazoxanide. What are the recommendations?

These combinations should never be used for two major reasons:
1. *Entamoeba histolytica* and helminthic infections are very rare in infants and young children as a cause of acute watery diarrhea.
2. Most of the fixed drug combinations are irrational and their pharmacodynamics is incompatible.

Q6. What is the indication for chemotherapeutic agents like metronidazole and nitazoxanide?

E. histolytica and giardiasis infections are rare in children. These agents should only be used when stool examination shows *E. histolytica* with ingested red blood cells (RBCs) or giardiasis. In few cases where bloody diarrhea does not respond to second-line of antibiotics like third-generation cephalosporins, metronidazole may be added.

Q7. What are the common bacterial causes of diarrhea with antibiotics of choice?

Common bacterial causes of diarrhea are:

- *E. coli, Shigella,* and *Salmonella*: Third-generation cephalosporins, quinolones, and co-trimoxazole
- *Vibrio cholerae*: Tetracycline, doxycycline, quinolones, and azithromycin
- *Campylobacter*: Azithromycin and quinolones
- *Listeria*: Ampicillin and co-trimoxazole.

Q8. Food poisoning is caused many times by *Salmonella* or *Staphylococcus*. What antibiotics should be used?

Most of the uncomplicated foodborne infections, although caused by bacterial contaminations of food, are self-limiting and may not require use of antibiotics. Antibiotics mainly oral, third-generation cephalosporins can be given in severely ill toxic child.

Q9. Why do you need antibiotics for travelers' diarrhea?

Almost 80% cases of travelers' diarrhea are due to bacterial pathogens mainly *E. coli* group. *Salmonella* and *Shigella* can also cause travelers' diarrhea. Hence, use of third-generation cephalosporins or quinolones is indicated, particularly in severe cases. Rifaximin is also very good drug for travelers' diarrhea.

Q10. What is antibiotic-associated diarrhea? Does it always need antibiotics in treatment?

Unwarranted use of broad-spectrum antibiotics has resulted in lot of cases of antibiotic-associated diarrhea. Broad-spectrum antibiotics cause alteration in gut friendly microbiota and this allows overgrowth of opportunistic organisms like *C. difficile* or fungi causing antibiotic-associated diarrhea. These diarrheas are severe in immunocompromised patients. Opportunistic organisms, particularly *C. difficile* and fungi are responsible for antibiotic-associated diarrhea.

In a culture or histopathology proven infections with *C. difficile,* oral vancomycin and metronidazole are the drugs of choice.

Q11. What are the factors affecting choice of antibiotics?

There are many factors on which the choice of antibiotics will depend. These are age, duration of infection, geographic location of patient, season, feeding history, nutritional status of patient, immune status of patients, severity of clinical conditions, duration of diarrhea, etc.

Q12. Should quinolones be used in pediatric age group?

Fluoroquinolones have a wide spectrum against variety of agents including *Shigella, Salmonella,* cholera, and *Campylobacter*. Because of arthropathic nature of the drug its use in pediatric age group is always under controversy. However, several studies have confirmed safety of ciprofloxacin use for this diarrhea in pediatric age group. Because of low cost, availability of liquid formulations and wide-spectrum against enteric pathogens quinolones has a place in management of acute diarrhea in poor countries like India.

Q13. Many western protocols suggest use of azithromycin for acute diarrhea? What is the status of azithromycin?

Although azithromycin has very high efficacy in majority of bacterial infections causing acute gastroenteritis (AGE) including *Shigella, Salmonella,* and *Campylobacter* as well as *E. coli*. Its routine use as first-line drug should be avoided for the fear of rapidly increasing resistance against the drug particularly in developing countries.

Q14. Choice of antibiotic according to causative organism.

Table 1 presents choice of antibiotic according to causative organism.

Table 1: Choice of antibiotic according to causative organism.

Organisms	*First-line drug*	*Alternative*
Campylobacter	Azithromycin	Ciprofloxacin, vancomycin
Clostridium difficile	Metronidazole	Vancomycin
Salmonella (nontyphoidal)	Amoxycillin, ceftriaxone	Co-trimoxazole
Shigella	Ceftriaxone, azithromycin	Cefixime, quinolone
V. cholerae	Doxycycline (>8 years)	Ciprofloxacin
E. coli	Cefixime, ceftriaxone, co-trimoxazole	Quinolone

Q15. What are the risk factors for pseudomembranous colitis?

Pseudomembranous colitis is a serious condition and it has certain risk factors.

- History of recent hospitalization with use of broad-spectrum antibiotics

- Use of gastric acid blockers
- Multiple comorbidities
- Inflammatory bowel disease (IBD)
- Immunocompromised host.

Clostridium difficile is the organism and metronidazole and vancomycin are drug of choice.

Q16. What are the indications of intravenous (IV) antibiotics?

In an uncomplicated patient oral antibiotics treatment is very effective, certain conditions require administration of IV antibiotics.

- Very toxic child in septicemia or shock
- Persistent vomiting
- Severe dehydration
- Severe acute malnutrition
- Patient with abdominal distention
- Patient with pneumonia and meningitis causing parenteral diarrhea.

Q17. What is campylobacter infection? What is the treatment?

Usually people get infection from food particularly under cooked poultry or sewage contaminated water. It causes diarrhea with mucus and abdominal pain. It may be self-limiting in healthy individuals but can cause morbidity in immunocompromised host.

Treatment of choice is azithromycin/erythromycin or quinolones.

Q18. Is antibiotic treatment a must for persistent diarrhea?

Persistent diarrhea is by definition a diarrhea beyond 14 days. By 14 days most of the viral diarrhea has stopped even without treatment, hence persistence of diarrhea beyond 14 days merits use of antibiotics in many cases.

Two most important reasons for persistent diarrhea:

- Malabsorption including lactose intolerance
- Subacute bacterial infection.

Common agents and therapies for persistent diarrhea are given in **Table 2**.

Table 2: Common agents and therapies for persistent diarrhea.

	First-line drug	***Alternative***
Giardiasis	Nitazoxanide	Metronidazole
Cryptosporidium	Paromomycin	Nitazoxanide
Cyclospora, E. Histolytica	Metronidazole	Tinidazole
Cytomegalovirus	Ganciclovir (5 mg/kg/day)	
Common intestinal bacterial infection	Already discussed	

Q19. Why antibiotics are required in a child with severe acute malnutrition (SAM)?

A SAM child has very low immunity and use of broad-spectrum antibiotics is suggested.

Rationale for antibiotics:

- High prevalence and risk of infection in SAM [like pneumonia, urinary tract infection (UTI), bacteremia]
- Diagnosis of infection clinically misleading as clinical manifestation of infection may not be apparent
- Severe acute malnutrition child have bacterial overgrowth in their small bowel (d/f, achlorhydria, low gut mobility, and impaired sugar absorption).

Q20. What is IAP recommendation of antibiotics use in SAM?

The IAP recommendation of antibiotic use in SAM child is as below.

- Ampicillin (IV × 2 days, oral × 5 days) + gentamycin/amikacin (×7 days)
- If not improve, add ceftriaxone
- If meningitis suspected go for lumbar puncture (LP) and start Ceftriaxone + amikacin × 14–21 days
- If staphylococcal infection is suspected add cloxacillin (100 mg/kg/day QD).

Q21. Is metronidazole indicated in diarrhea in patient with SAM?

Some studies suggested that it should be given:

- 45% of SAM with chronic diarrhea—giardiasis
- 27% of SAM without diarrhea—Giardiasis
- Active against bacterial overgrowth
- High incidence of anaerobic infection.

Q22. What are the indications of antibiotic therapy in HIV?

- Child on inadequate/no ARI or CD4 less than 500—ciprofloxacin + metronidazole
- If poor response × 5–7 days go for stool for ova, cyst, and protozoa for at least three times, add co-trimoxazole to ciprofloxacin + metronidazole
- If no response for 7 days go for sigmoidoscopy with biopsy for *Cytomegalovirus* or *Campylobacter*
- *Cryptosporidium* should be treated with nitazoxanide
- *Cytomegalovirus*—ganciclovir (12 mg/kg/day BD ×6 weeks).

Q23. What are the organisms causing diarrhea in HIV patient and their drugs of choice?

- Common organisms in HIV are *E. histolytic* and *Giardia lamblia*
- *Cryptosporidium*: Nitazoxanide or azithromycin
- *Microsporidia*: Albendazole 7.5 mg/kg/dose × BD or nitazoxanide
- *Isospora*: Cotrimoxazole 5 mg/kg/dose QD ×10 days then BD × 3 days or
- Pyrimethamine (if an allergic of trimethoprim sulfa drug)
- *Cyclospora*: Co-trimoxazole 5 mg/kg/dose BD × 7 days.

Q24. What is the treatment of cholera?

Rehydration is the first priority in the treatment of cholera. The goal of the rehydration phase is to restore normal hydration status, which should take no more than 4 hours. In conjunction with hydration, treatment with antibiotics is recommended for severely or moderately dehydrated children who continue to pass a large volume of stool during rehydration treatment. Antibiotic choices should be guided by local antibiotic susceptibility patterns. In most countries, doxycycline is recommended as first-line treatment for adults and children above 8 years, while azithromycin is recommended as first-line treatment for children and pregnant women. Treatment with a single dose of doxycycline (3–4 mg/kg) has shown to be equivalent to tetracycline treatment. Doxycycline is equally effective clinically in lessening the diarrhea; the duration of excretion of the *Vibrio*, however, is not as effectively shortened as with tetracycline therapy. During an epidemic or outbreak, antibiotic susceptibility should be monitored through regular testing of sample isolates from various geographic areas.

CHAPTER 15

Urinary Tract Infection

Upendra Kinjawadekar, Vipin Goyal

Q1. What is urinary tract infection (UTI)?

An infection in any part of the urinary system, i.e. urethra, bladder, ureter or kidneys, is called a UTI. These infections can be mostly found involving the lower urinary tract bladder and urethra.

Q2. What are the causative organisms?

- *Gram-negative bacteria*: *Escherichia coli* (most common), *Klebsiella, Proteus, Enterobacter,* and *Citrobacter.*
- *Gram-positive bacteria*: *Staphylococcus saprophyticus, Enterococcus,* and rarely, *Staphylococcus aureus.*

Q3. How to diagnose UTI?

Urinary tract infection can be suspected based on findings on urinalysis or symptoms or both. Urine culture is necessary for confirmation and appropriate therapy.

Q4. When to start empirical therapy for UTI?

Early and aggressive empirical therapy is necessary to prevent renal damage. Early therapy is indicated in:

- Fever (>39°C or > 48 hours)
- Ill appearance
- Costovertebral angle tenderness
- Known immune deficiency
- Known urologic abnormality.

Q5. What is the choice of agent for UTI?

Empiric therapy for UTI should include an antibiotic that covers *E. coli.* The antibiotic of choice is guided by local resistance patterns.

Around 50% of *E. coli* are resistant to amoxicillin or ampicillin. In addition, there is increasing resistance to first-generation cephalosporins (cephalexin), amoxicillin-clavulanate, ampicillin-sulbactam, and trimethoprim-sulfamethoxazole (TMP-SMX) in some communities.

Third-generation cephalosporins (cefixime, cefpodoxime, and ceftriaxone) and aminoglycosides (gentamicin and amikacin) are appropriate first-line agents for empiric treatment of UTI in children.

These drugs are not sufficient in patients in whom *Enterococcus* UTI is suspected, like children with instrumentation of urinary tract or anatomical abnormality. In such patients, amoxicillin or ampicillin should be added.

Q6. What are the antibiotics used for oral therapy?

Most children older than 2 months of age who are not vomiting can be treated with oral antibiotics. The agent of choice is cefixime (16 mg/kg OD on day1, followed by 8 mg/kg OD to complete therapy) for 14 days.

Other cephalosporins that may be used for oral therapy include:

- Cefdinir (14 mg/kg/d OD)
- Ceftibuten (9 mg/kg OD)
- Cefpodoxime (10 mg/kg/d divided into two doses).

Fluoroquinolones (ciprofloxacin) are effective against *E. coli*, but not routinely used as first-line agents. They are used for UTIs caused by *Pseudomonas aeruginosa*. The prevalence of extended-spectrum beta-lactamase (ESBL) producing gram-negative organisms is increasing in many parts and the clinician must know the local prevalence.

Nitrofurantoin and nalidixic acid do not have sufficient parenchymal or serum concentration and therefore should not be used to treat febrile UTI or urosepsis.

Q7. What are the antibiotics used for inpatient parenteral therapy?

Oral antibiotics are as good as parenteral in most clinical situations. However in hospital, parenteral therapy is indicated in children with:

- Vomiting or inability to tolerate oral medications
- Very young infant (<2 months)
- Clinical urosepsis
- Lack of outpatient follow-up
- Failure to respond to outpatient therapy.

Cephalosporins and aminoglycosides are appropriate first-line therapy for empiric treatment of UTI in children. Definitive therapy is based on the results of urine culture and sensitivities. Ampicillin should be included if enterococcal UTI is suspected. The doses are as follows:

- Ampicillin [100 mg/kg/day intravenous (IV) in four divided doses]
- Gentamicin (7.5 mg/kg/day IV in three divided doses)
- Amikacin (15 mg/kg/day single dose)
- Cefotaxime (150 mg/kg/day IV in three or four divided doses)
- Ceftriaxone (50–75 mg/kg/day IV)
- Cefepime (100 mg/kg/day IV divided in two doses).

Parenteral therapy is to be continued until the patient is clinically improved and able to tolerate oral liquids and medications.

Q8. What are the antibiotics used for outpatient parenteral therapy?
Once daily parenteral administration of gentamicin/amikacin or ceftriaxone in a day treatment center may avoid the need for hospital admission in select patients.

Q9. What are the antibiotics used for children with recent antibiotic exposure or recurrent UTI?
Pending culture and sensitivity results, antibiotics from a different class should be used for empirical therapy, after reviewing the antimicrobial susceptibilities of the most recent urinary pathogens.

Q10. How is the response to antibiotic therapy assessed?
Usually the clinical condition of most patients improves within 24–48 hours of initiating the appropriate antimicrobial therapy. In those patients whose condition worsens or fails to improve as expected within 48 hours, a renal and bladder ultrasonography should be performed (if not done before) and broadening antimicrobial therapy is indicated depending upon the results of culture and sensitivity report. A pediatric nephrologist's opinion should be sought in patients with recurrent UTI, complicated UTI, and UTI with underlying urogenital anomaly.

Q11. When should prophylactic antibiotics be used?
Though antibiotic prophylaxis reduces chances of recurrence by half, whether it prevents renal scarring is controversial. Hence, the decision to put a child on prophylactic antibiotics who do not have vesicoureteral reflux (VUR) should be case based (e.g. those with single kidney, renal abscess or bladder bowel dysfunction) after discussing with the parents.

Indian Society of Pediatric Nephrology recommends prophylactic antibiotics for UTI below 1 year of age while awaiting culture results, those with VUR and frequent febrile UTIs (three or more episodes in a year even if urinary tract is normal). Following antibiotics are used for prophylaxis at 30% of the therapeutic dose:

- Trimethoprim-sulfamethoxazole
- Amoxicillin
- Cephalexin
- Nitrofurantoin.

CHAPTER 16

Enteric Fever

Parang N Mehta

Q1. What causes enteric fever?

Salmonella typhi/paratyphi A/B/C (now termed as *Salmonella enterica serotype typhi or Salmonella enterica serotype paratyphi),* a gram-negative bacillus, are the infecting organisms. Infections due to *S. typhi* (typhoid fever) are the most common, but with increasing immunization coverage with the typhoid Vi vaccine, cases of paratyphoid fever (*S. paratyphi A*) are on the rise. Few cases are caused by *S. paratyphi B*. There is also a variety called *S. paratyphi C,* but it is seen only in the far East.

Q2. Is this disease common in children?

Yes, children are the major sufferers. Around the world, the age group of 5–15 years has the peak incidence. In India, however, children of the age group 2–5 years also have a high incidence. Recently many cases of typhoid fever are seen in children below 2 years and in infancy also. Mortality is also higher in children, compared to adolescents and adults.

Q3. What is the pattern of antimicrobial resistance in *S. typhi/paratyphi?*

Introduction of chloramphenicol as the antibiotic for *S. typhi* in the 1940s was followed by development of resistance to it within the next 2 years. Towards the end of the 1980s and the 1990s, *S. typhi* developed resistance to all the drugs that were then used as first-line antibiotic (chloramphenicol, trimethoprim, sulfamethoxazole, and ampicillin). Fluoroquinolones were introduced in the late 1980s and produced good results. However, over the past decade there has been a progressive increase in the minimum inhibitory concentrations (MICs) of ciprofloxacin in *S. typhi* and *S. paratyphi*. Since the current MICs are still below the National Committee for Clinical Laboratory Standards (NCCLS) susceptibility breakpoint, laboratory reports will continue to report *S. typhi/paratyphi* as ciprofloxacin/ofloxacin sensitive. But use of fluoroquinolones in this scenario is associated with a high incidence of clinical failure. It has been demonstrated that resistance to nalidixic acid is a surrogate marker for high ciprofloxacin MICs and predicts fluoroquinolone failure. Third-generation cephalosporins, ceftrixone and cefixime are now used as first-line agents for therapy of enteric fever. The strain of extensively drug-resistant (XDR), *S. enterica* serovar Typhi is resistant to five classes of antibiotics (chloramphenicol, ampicillin, trimethoprim-sulfamethoxazole, fluoroquinolones, and third-generation cephalosporins) and is responsible for an outbreak in Pakistan that began in November 2016.

Q4. Should blood cultures be routinely done before starting treatment?

Culture of *S. typhi/paratyphi* is the gold standard for diagnosis, and has a specificity of 100%. More importantly, it will guide us about the drug sensitivity and resistance of the organism. In this time of multidrug resistance, blood culture is an investigation of choice and will be cost-effective in long run and will prevent antibiotic abuse.

Q5. What are the treatment options for uncomplicated typhoid fever?

In endemic areas most of the typhoid cases can be managed at home with proper oral antibiotics and good nursing care. Close medical follow-up is necessary to look for development of complications or failure to respond to therapy.

Treatment of uncomplicated enteric fever includes third-generation cephalosporin, cefixime, in a dose of 20 mg/kg/day for 14 days. Alternatively, azithromycin in a dose of 15 mg/kg/day for 7 days is also recommended as a second like drug.

Q6. What is the treatment for enteric fever in hospitalized children?

All severe typhoid cases should be hospitalized. Children who are too sick to eat and drink adequately, or are vomiting frequently, should be hospitalized. Treatment of severe typhoid fever includes parenteral ceftriaxone, 100 mg/kg/day followed by oral switch to cefixime once the child improve and tolerates orally. In exceptional cases, with severe allergic reactions to ceftriaxone, aztreonam, 50–100 mg/kg/day for 10–14 days is advised.

Q7. If the patient does not respond to first-line drugs, what are second-line drugs?

For oral use, the second-line drug is azithromycin (20 mg/kg/day). For enteric fever, this drug must be given for 7 days. The child that cannot tolerate oral drugs should be given aztreonam (50–100 mg/kg/day). This drug also should be given for 14 days.

Q8. Should we combine two antibiotics to deal with nonresponse?

Being an intracellular pathogen, enteric fever responds slowly to treatment. Even with parenteral ceftriaxone, it is usual for defervescence to take

5–7 days. Resistance to third-generation cephalosporins is very rare and adding another drug does not give significant clinical benefit.

If the child remains febrile and toxic for longer than expected, think of complication, other peripheral causes like phlebitis, immune-mediated fever, serious situation like hemophagocytic lymphohistiocytosis (HLH) and lastly drug resistance. By this time, the culture and sensitivity report should be available to guide further therapy. It is very important to send blood cultures before starting antibiotic therapy.

Q9. What is the treatment of relapses?

If the child responded to a drug at the first instance, the drug will be effective again. The same drug should be given for the full course. There is no need to change the effective drug.

Q10. Are the older drugs chloramphenicol, ampicillin, and co-trimoxazole effective again currently?

A proportion of culture reports show the organism to be sensitive to some or all these drugs. However, this cannot be known in advance and these drugs cannot be used empirically as first-line therapy. The risk of failed therapy is currently unacceptably high with these antibiotics.

If first-line therapy fails and the culture report shows sensitivity to ampicillin or co-trimoxazole, they can be used. Chloramphenicol should not be used because of the danger of fatal aplastic anemia.

FURTHER READING

1. CIDRAP. (2018). XDR typhoid in Pakistan carries added resistance genes. [online] Available from http://www.cidrap.umn.edu/news-perspective/2018/02/study-xdr-typhoid-pakistan-carries-added-resistance-genes [Accessed December 2018].

CHAPTER 17

Spontaneous Bacterial Peritonitis

Bhaskar Shenoy

Q1. How do you define spontaneous bacterial peritonitis (SBP)?
Spontaneous bacterial peritonitis is defined as an ascitic fluid infection without an evident intra-abdominal surgically treatable source. In other words, it is an infection of ascitic fluid without an apparent source.

Q2. Describe the pathogenesis of SBP?
One of the early steps in the development of SBP is a disturbance in gut flora with overgrowth and extraintestinal dissemination of a specific organism, most commonly *Escherichia coli*. Cirrhosis predisposes to the development of bacterial overgrowth, possibly because of altered small intestinal motility and the presence of hypochlorhydria due to use of proton pump inhibitors. In addition, patients with cirrhosis may have increased intestinal permeability. Whether or not they are present in increased numbers, bacteria within the gut lumen can traverse the intestinal wall and colonize mesenteric lymph nodes. This phenomenon is called translocation. Bacterial ascites can occur if the lymphatic channel carrying contaminated lymph ruptures because of the high flow and high pressure associated with portal hypertension. Alternatively, the organism can move from the mesenteric lymphatics to the systemic circulation and then percolate through the liver and weep across Glisson's capsule to enter the ascitic fluid.

Q3. What are the clinical manifestations of SBP?
Manifestations may include fever, malaise, and symptoms of ascites and worsening hepatic failure. SBP is particularly common in cirrhotic ascites. This infection can cause serious sequelae or death. Patients have symptoms and signs of ascites.

Signs of SBP may also include encephalopathy, worsening hepatic failure, and unexplained clinical deterioration. Peritoneal signs (e.g. abdominal tenderness and rebound) are present but may be somewhat diminished by the presence of ascitic fluid. In addition, patients with ascites admitted to the hospital for other reasons should also undergo paracentesis to look for evidence of SBP. A low clinical suspicion for SBP does not obviate the need for testing.

Fever: Fever is the most common clinical manifestation of SBP. It is important to appreciate that patients with advanced cirrhosis are usually mildly hypothermic.

Abdominal pain and tenderness: Diffuse abdominal pain is the hallmark of peritonitis. However, the pain can be very subtle in SBP due to the presence of ascites and some patients are asymptomatic. The pain is usually diffuse and continuous; it is different from the pain induced by stretching of the abdominal wall due to tense ascites.

As with abdominal pain, abdominal tenderness is a classic sign of peritonitis that can be subtle in SBP. These patients do not develop a rigid abdomen, although rebound tenderness may be present in advanced cases.

Altered mental status: The clinical sign of infection that is frequently overlooked in the patient with cirrhosis is a subtle change in mental status. While the patient may present with frank delirium, confusion, or cognitive slowing, the alteration in mental status may be so subtle. Both the infection itself and hepatic decompensation may contribute to this problem.

Diarrhea: Diarrhea is common in patients with SBP. An alteration in gut flora with overgrowth of one organism (usually *E. coli*) is the possible explanation.

Paralytic ileus, hypotension, and hypothermia: These more severe signs are indicative of advanced infection and a poor likelihood of survival. It is important to detect infection and begin antibiotic treatment before this stage is reached.

Q4. What are the organisms causing SBP?

The most common bacteria causing SBP are gram-negative *E. coli, Klebsiella pneumoniae,* and gram-positive *Streptococcus pneumoniae.* Usually only a single organism is involved.

Q5. What are the risk factors for SBP?

The vast majority of patients with SBP have advanced cirrhosis. SBP can be a complication of nephrotic syndrome. Other risk factors (most of which are associated with cirrhosis) include:

- Ascitic fluid total protein concentration less than 1 g/dL
- Prior episode of SBP
- Serum total bilirubin concentration above 2.5 mg/dL
- Variceal hemorrhage
- Malnutrition
- Use of proton pump inhibitors.

The combination of certain clinical and laboratory features is also associated with an increased risk of SBP.

- An ascitic fluid total protein less than 1.5 g/dL (<15 g/L) with
- Child–Pugh score more than or equal to 9 points with serum bilirubin more than or equal to 3 mg/dL or with
- Plasma creatinine more than or equal to 1.2 mg/dL, blood urea nitrogen more than or equal to 25 mg/dL or plasma sodium less than or equal to 130 mEq/L.

Q6. What is the importance of early recognition of SBP?

It is important to recognize SBP early in the course of infection because there is frequently a very short window of opportunity during which to intervene to ensure a good outcome. If the opportunity is missed, shock ensues, followed rapidly by multisystem organ failure. Survival is unlikely in patients who develop shock prior to initiation of empiric antibiotics. One report estimated that survival decreased by approximately 8% for each hour of delay in starting of antibiotics in patients with septic shock.

Q7. How do we confirm the diagnosis?

- Diagnostic paracentesis
- Diagnosis requires a high index of suspicion and liberal use of diagnostic paracentesis, including culture. Transferring ascitic fluid to blood culture media before incubation increases the sensitivity of culture to almost 70%. Polymorphonuclear (PMN) leukocyte count of more than 250 cells/μL is diagnostic of SBP. Blood cultures are also indicated. Because SBP usually results from a single organism, finding mixed flora on culture suggests a perforated abdominal viscus or contaminated specimen.

Q8. How to interpret the ascitic fluid in traumatic paracentesis?

- One potential source of error in the PMN count is that hemorrhage into the ascitic fluid, as in a traumatic paracentesis, leads to red cell and white cell entry into the fluid. A corrected PMN count should be calculated if there is bloody fluid.
- One PMN is subtracted from the absolute PMN count for every 250 red cells/mm^3 PMNs lyse rapidly, much more so than red cells. Thus, if the bleeding episode occurred prior to (rather than during) paracentesis, the PMNs that entered the fluid may have lysed, and the corrected PMN count may be a negative number.

Q9. How do you differentiate between SBP and secondary bacterial peritonitis?

The distinction of SBP from secondary bacterial peritonitis is based largely upon ascitic fluid analysis, imaging studies, and the response to treatment.

Two varieties of secondary bacterial peritonitis have been reported: perforation peritonitis (e.g. perforated peptic ulcer into ascites) and nonperforation peritonitis (e.g. perinephric abscess).

The distinction of secondary bacterial peritonitis from SBP is crucial because of the importance of appropriate therapy:

- *Clinical signs and symptoms*: The signs and symptoms of both SBP and surgical peritonitis in the presence of ascites can be surprisingly subtle. Ascites prevents the development of a rigid abdomen by separating the visceral from the parietal peritoneal surfaces.
- *Ascitic fluid analysis*: The initial (pretreatment) ascitic fluid analysis can be extremely helpful in determining the degree of suspicion of secondary bacterial peritonitis. Proposed laboratory criteria for diagnosis of secondary bacterial peritonitis (sometimes referred to as Runyon's criteria) include at least two of the following ascitic fluid findings:
  - Total protein more than 1 g/dL (10 g/L)
  - Glucose less than 50 mg/dL (2.8 mmol/L)
  - Lactate dehydrogenase (LDH) more than the upper limit of normal for serum.
- *Imaging studies*: Patients who meet the criteria for secondary bacterial peritonitis should undergo emergency plain and upright abdominal films and a computed tomographic scan of the abdomen. Emergency laparotomy should be performed if free air or a surgically treatable source of infection is documented.

Q10. How do we treat SBP?

Any cirrhotic patient with a positive ascitic fluid culture who has concerning signs or symptoms that may indicate infection, such as fever (temperature greater than 37.8°C or 100° F), abdominal pain, or unexplained hepatic encephalopathy, should receive empiric antibiotic treatment for spontaneous bacterial peritonitis, regardless of ascitic fluid PMN count. Broad-spectrum antibiotic therapy is recommended for treatment of proven or suspected SBP and may be narrowed when susceptibility results become available. If SBP is diagnosed, an antibiotic such as cefotaxime 100 mg/kg q 8 hours (pending Gram stain and culture results) is given for at least 5 days and until ascitic fluid shows less than 250 PMNs/μL. Antibiotics increase the chance of survival. Cefotaxime given intravenously has been shown to produce excellent ascitic fluid levels. Because SBP recurs within a year in up to 70% of patients, prophylactic antibiotics are indicated.

Antibiotic prophylaxis in ascitic patients with variceal hemorrhage decreases the risk of SBP.

Indications for antibiotic therapy: Empiric therapy for SBP should be started in a patient with ascites who has one or more of the following findings:

- Temperature greater than 37.8°C (100°F)
- Abdominal pain and/or tenderness
- A change in mental status
- Ascitic fluid PMN count more than or equal to 250 cells/mm^3.

Secondary bacterial peritonitis is often a polymicrobial diseases and hence combination of third generation cephalosporin with metronidazole is indicated.Alternatively cefpoperazone with sulbactam is also advocted. Extended spectrum antibiotics, such as Pipracillin-tazobactam or carbapenems, may even be considered in serious nosocomial cases and/or very serious and sick patients.. The choice of treatment will depend on location of acquisition (community versus nosocomial), local resistance patterns, and culture sensitivity results when available. The following summarizes recommended and commonly used antimicrobial regimens to treat SBP.

Q11. What is the prognosis of SBP?

The infection-related mortality from SBP is low with appropriate treatment. Several reports found no infection-related deaths if treatment was started prior to shock or frank renal failure.

In patients who have developed septic shock, mortality is high, but early initiation of appropriate antimicrobial therapy is associated with improved outcomes. Liver transplantation should be seriously considered for survivors of SBP who are otherwise good transplantation candidates.

Q12. What is the role of prophylaxis in SBP?

Antibiotic prophylaxis for patients with risk factors for SBP (including ascitic fluid protein concentration less than 1 g/dL, variceal hemorrhage, or a prior episode of SBP) decreases the risk of bacterial infection and mortality. *The usual antibiotics used in prophylaxis are trimethoprim-sulfamethoxazole and fluoroquinolones.*

Guidelines suggest that antibiotic prophylaxis should be given to the following patients:

- Patients with cirrhosis and gastrointestinal bleeding. Antibiotic prophylaxis in this setting has been shown to decrease mortality in randomized trials.
- Patients who have had one or more episodes of SBP. In such patients, recurrence rates of SBP within 1 year have been reported to be close to 70%.

- Patients with cirrhosis and ascites if the ascitic fluid protein is less than 1.5 g/dL (15 g/L) along with either impaired renal function or liver failure.

In addition, antibiotic prophylaxis to patients with cirrhosis who are hospitalized for other reasons and have an ascitic protein concentration of less than 1 g/dL (10 g/L).

Q13. What are the general measures to be followed in the management of SBP?

These measures include:

- Diuretic therapy. Diuresis concentrates ascitic fluid, thereby raising ascitic fluid opsonic activity, which may help prevent SBP.
- Early recognition and aggressive treatment of localized infections (e.g. cystitis and cellulitis). This can help to prevent bacteremia and SBP.
- Restricting use of proton pump inhibitors. Proton pump inhibitor use has been associated with an increased risk of SBP in many (but not all) studies. As a result, proton pump inhibitors should only be given to patients who have clear indications for their use.

CHAPTER 18

Skin and Soft Tissue Infections and Necrotizing Fasciitis

Abhay K Shah

Q1. Which are the common bacterial skin infections?

Skin and soft-tissue infections (SSTIs) are best described according to the anatomical site of infection.

- Impetigo involving epidermis
- Folliculitis—a superficial pustular infection involving the hair follicle and perifollicular structure
- Furuncles—single hair follicle associated infections extending through the dermis into the subcutaneous tissue
- Carbuncles involve several adjacent hair follicles forming a coalescent mass
- Erysipelas involves the upper dermis including the superficial lymphatics
- Cellulitis diffuse skin infection that involves the deep dermis and subcutaneous fat tissues
- Necrotizing SSTI involving fascia, muscles and deeper tissue.

Q2. Which are the common etiological agents for SSTIs?

The vast majority of SSTIs are caused by *Staphylococcus aureus* and beta-hemolytic streptococci, usually Lancefield groups A, C, and G with group B occurring in diabetics and the elderly. Localized pus-producing lesions such as boils, abscesses, carbuncles, and localized wound sepsis are usually staphylococcal, while rapidly spreading infections such as erysipelas, lymphangitis or cellulitis are usually caused by beta-hemolytic streptococci.

Gram-negative and anaerobic bacteria are more common in association with surgical site infections of the abdominal wall or infections of the soft tissue in the anal and perineal region. Polymicrobial infections involving both gram-positive and gram-negative organisms occur particularly where tissue vascular perfusion is compromised, such as diabetic foot infection or infection of ischemic or venous ulcers.

Q3. What are the common risk factors for SSTIs and their recurrence?

- Poor hygiene
- Eczema and allergic dermatosis

- Recurrent hospital admissions
- Contact sports
- History of known contact with recurrent methicillin-resistant *S. aureus* (MRSA) or methicillin-susceptible *S. aureus* (MSSA) boils and abscesses
- Diabetes mellitus
- Immunocompromised child
- Steroids and immunosuppressive drugs
- Peripheral ischemic vascular diseases
- Drug addicts in adolescents.

Q4. What do you mean by complicated SSTIs?

Skin and soft-tissue infections accompanied by signs and symptoms of systemic toxicity such as fever, hypothermia/hyperpyrexia, tachycardia, and hypotension can be classified as complicated. They usually require hospitalization and surgical consultation.

Q5. How will you treat impetigo?

It is a common superficial skin infection characterized by inflammation and infection in the epidermis. This infection is primarily caused by *S. aureus* and *S. pyogenes* either alone or in combination.

It exists in two major forms; bullous impetigo and nonbullous impetigo (impetigo contagiosa).

- In case of minor lesions which is often self-limiting, simple measures like debridement of the crust with warm soak along with cleaning several times daily with antibacterial soap is adequate.
- In limited lesion, topical therapy with mupirocin application twice a day for 5 days is helpful
- Antibiotic therapy for impetigo should be a 7-day regimen with an agent active against *S. aureus* and streptococci because *S. aureus* isolates from impetigo and ecthyma are usually methicillin susceptible, oral cephalexin or cefadroxil is sufficient.
- When MRSA is suspected or confirmed, doxycycline, clindamycin, or sulfamethoxazole-trimethoprim (SMX-TMP) is recommended.
- Personal hygiene should be encouraged.

Q6. How will you manage folliculitis, furuncles, and carbuncles?

- In immunocompetent children folliculitis and small furuncles resolve spontaneously with use of warm compress and topical antibiotic therapy like mupirocin.
- Incision and drainage is needed for carbuncles and larger furuncles. Gram stain and culture of the pus or exudates from skin lesions are recommended to help identify the microbial agent.

- Systemic antibiotics should be reserved for children who have systemic signs such as fever, tachypnea, tachycardia or if associated cellulitis is present. Cephalexin or cefadroxil are the preferred agent for systemic usage. An antibiotic active against MRSA is recommended for patients with carbuncles or abscesses who have failed initial antibiotic treatment or have markedly impaired host defenses or in patients with systemic inflammatory response syndrome (SIRS) and hypotension.
- In repeated attacks of furunculosis, to eradicate staphylococcal carriage application of mupirocin ointment twice daily in the anterior nares for the first 5 days of each month is recommended to reduce the recurrence by half.

Q7. What are microbes causing cellulitis and erysipelas? How will you manage?

Streptococcus pyogenes is the most frequently responsible for cellulitis, but *S. aureus* is also an important cause in children usually those associated with abscess or other primary lesion. *Haemophilus influenzae* and *Streptococcus pneumoniae* can also cause cellulitis in young children.

The treatment of cellulitis and erysipelas requires systemic antibiotics active against both streptococci and staphylococci. Suitable agents include cloxacillin, cephalexin, clindamycin or co-amoxiclav for 5–7 days. Cefazolin or anti-staphylococcal penicillin like cloxacillin is recommended for definitive therapy of lesions caused by MSSA. For patients whose cellulitis is associated with penetrating trauma, evidence of MRSA infection elsewhere, nasal colonization with MRSA, injection drug use, or SIRS, vancomycin or another antimicrobial effective against both MRSA and streptococci is recommended. Elevation of the affected area hastens recovery by aiding drainage of edema.

Q8. When will you admit the patient with cellulitis?

Hospitalization is recommended if there is concern for a deeper necrotizing infection, for patients with poor adherence to therapy, for patient with systemic toxemia, for infection in a severely immunocompromised patient, or if outpatient treatment is failing.

Q9. What is necrotizing SSTI?

This medicosurgical emergency is a life-threatening and invasive. Soft-tissue infection caused by aggressive, usually gas-forming bacteria, which primarily involves the superficial fascia and extends rapidly along subcutaneous tissue planes with relative sparing of skin and underlying muscle.

Q10. What would be the clinical presentation in a case of necrotizing fasciitis?

Clinical presentation includes fever, signs of systemic toxicity, and pain out of proportion to the clinical findings. The diagnosis of fasciitis may not be apparent upon first seeing the patient. Overlying cutaneous inflammation may resemble cellulitis.

However, features that suggest involvement of deeper tissues include:

- Severe pain that seems disproportionate to the clinical findings
- Failure to respond to initial antibiotic therapy
- The hard, wooden feel of the subcutaneous tissue, extending beyond the area of apparent skin involvement
- Edema or tenderness extending beyond the cutaneous erythema
- Crepitus, indicating gas in the tissues
- Skin necrosis or ecchymoses
- Systemic toxicity, often with altered mental status.

The most important diagnostic criteria is the appearance of subcutaneous tissue at the operating table. The subcutaneous tissue is swollen, has dull gray appearance with dish water fluid like discharge from the affected area.

Q11. Which are the types of necrotizing fasciitis?

Necrotizing fasciitis is empirically divided into two categories based on number of organisms involved; monomicrobial and polymicrobial.

Monomicrobial is more common; usually caused by *S. pyogenes* or *S. aureus*. Other organisms like *Vibrio vulnificus*, anaerobic streptococci and *Aeromonas hydrophila* may also be responsible. Fasciitis occurring after trivial injuries or chickenpox are almost always due to *S. pyogenes* and very rarely due to community-associated MRSA.

Polymicrobial forms are less common and mainly caused by both aerobic and anaerobic bacteria. Common isolates include *Streptococcus* other than group A, *S. aureus, Enterococcus, E. coli, Bacteroides, Clostridia,* and *Peptostreptococcus*. Most of them originate from the bowel flora and follow surgical procedures involving the gut or penetrating abdominal trauma.

Q12. How will you manage a case of necrotizing fasciitis?

- In addition to stabilization of patient with maintenance of airway, breathing, and circulation the first and foremost in the treatment of necrotizing fasciitis is the immediate institution of definitive treatment without any delay for investigations.
- Surgical debridement is the mainstay of therapy and at times repeated debridement by the surgical team may be warranted.
- Antibiotic therapy should be aimed at the most likely pathogen(s) responsible and is required till there is obvious clinical improvement. Empiric treatment of necrotizing fasciitis should include agents effective against both aerobes, including MRSA and anaerobes.

- Empirically for polymicrobial disease vancomycin, or linezolid, or daptomycin combined with piperacillin-tazobactam, or a carbapenem (imipenem-cilastatin, meropenem or ertapenem), or ceftriaxone plus metronidazole should be started. Once the microbial etiology has been determined, the antibiotic coverage should be modified.
- For monomicrobial infection ceftriaxone along with clindamycin should be used. Clindamycin suppresses toxin and cytokine production.
- For MSSA, cloxacillin or cefazolin may be used.
- For MRSA, vancomycin or linezolid is the drug of choice.
- Additional studies of the efficacy of intravenous immunoglobulin (IVIG) are necessary before a recommendation can be made supporting its use.

Q13. Mention antibiotic choices with dosage for SSIT.

- Cloxacillin 50–100 mg/kg/day in four divided doses
- Cephalexin 25–50 mg/kg/day in four divided doses
- Cefazolin 50 mg/kg in three divided doses
- Clindamycin (if local strains susceptible) 10–20 mg/kg/day in three divided doses
- Amoxicillin/clavulanate 40 mg/kg/day of the amoxicillin component in two divided doses.

Q14. Which are anti-MRSA drugs? Drugs for MRSA?

- Doxycycline (bacteriostatic, for children 100 mg BD older than 7 years)
- TMP-SMX 8–12 mg/kg (based on trimethoprim component) in either four divided doses IV or two divided doses PO
- Vancomycin 40–60 mg/kg/day IV 6–8 hourly (IV infusion over 1 hour or more)
- Linezolid 30 mg/kg/day PO or IV q8 hourly
- Clindamycin 10–20 mg/kg/day in three divided doses PO
- Daptomycin (no pediatric data) 4 mg/kg/day OD × 7 days.

FURTHER READING

1. Abhay K. Shah, Skin and Soft tissue infetions. Indian Journal of Practical Pediatrics 2015;17(40):275.
2. Liu C, Bayer A, Cosgrove SE, et al. Clinical Practice by the Infectious Diseases Society of America for the Treatment of Methicillin-Resistant *Staphylococcus aureus* Infections in Adults and Children. Clin Infect Dis. 2011;52(3):e18-e55.
3. Parthasarathy A. Textbook on Pediatric Infectious diseases, 2nd edition. New Delhi: Jaypee Brothers Medical Publishers (P) Ltd.; 2013.
4. Stevens DL, Bisno AL, Chambers HF, et al. Practice Guidelines for the Diagnosis and Management of Skin and Soft Tissue Infections: 2014 Update by the Infectious Diseases Society of America. Clin Infect Dis. 2014;59(2):e10-e52.

CHAPTER 19

Septic Arthritis

Ketan H Shah

Q1. Why it is important to diagnose and treat septic arthritis early?

If the condition is not diagnosed early, it has the potential to damage the synovium, adjacent cartilage, bone, and can cause permanent disability of affected part.

Q2. Which are the common organisms responsible for septic arthritis?

- *Staphylococcus aureus* is the most common in early age. *Haemophilus influenzae* is responsible for more than half of the cases. However, due to availability of vaccine, incidence has reduced significantly. Other bacteria includes *Streptococcus* group A and *Streptococcus pneumoniae.* Its incidence has also reduced due to vaccination. *Kingella kingae* is now recognized as the common agent after *S. aureus*.
- In sexually abused adolescent, gonococci are one important organism.
- Fungal infection as a cause in disseminated disease and in immunocompromised host. *Candida* can complicate systemic infection in newborn.
- Primary viral infections may have direct joint involvement or can cause reactive arthritis, e.g. parvovirus, rubella virus, and mumps virus. It can be immune-mediated or as postinfectious disease.
- Tuberculosis can cause acute, subacute (Pott's spine) or reactive arthritis termed as Poncet disease.
- Following gastrointestinal or urinary tract infection reactive arthritis can occur (*Salmonella, Shigella,* and *Enterobacteriaceae*).
- Lyme disease in western world is common etiological agent.
- Rickettsia and brucellosis can cause acute arthritis. Associated clinical features will give clue to the diagnosis.

Q3. Which are the common mechanisms for developing septic arthritis?

- Hematogenous seeding of the synovial space is the most common mechanism. Synovial membrane has a rich vascular supply and lacks basement membrane providing ideal environment for bacterial growth. Synovial and cartilage damage occurs due to action of inflammatory mediators.

- Direct inoculation.
- Contagious extension from an adjacent site.
- Overgrowth of skin flora.

Q4. Which joint is most commonly affected?

Knee joint is commonly affected. Hip, ankle, elbow, and shoulder joints are affected in descending order. Sometimes multiple joints are affected.

Q5. What are the clinical manifestations?

Most septic arthritis is monoarticular. Signs and symptoms differ depending upon the age and site of involvement.

Neonate: Irritability, fever, and difficult in moving limb are common symptoms. In neonates adjacent osteomyelitis is common.

Older infant would have fever, pain, decreased joint movement, and swelling. When lower limb involvement occurs limping is common presentation. In case of arthritis near long bones metaphysical involvement is commonly seen as metaphysis extends intra-articularly.

Sacroiliitis can be diagnosed by FABER maneuver. It is a maneuver that elicits pain during **F**lexion, **Ab**duction, and **E**xternal **R**otation of the hip joint. It detects pyogenic sacroiliitis.

Q6. What are the diagnostic tests?

- *Blood*: Blood culture is essential before giving antibiotic. Total white blood cell count, erythrocyte sedimentation rate (ESR), and C-reactive protein (CRP) are elevated in acute stage.
- *Joint aspiration*: It is a useful investigation. Findings are described in Table 1. However, these findings are not diagnostic. In hip aspiration fluid if counts are not found to be high than associated pyomyositis should be suspected and investigated. Gram-stain, Ziehl-Neelsen (ZN) stain, bacterial culture, cartridge-based nucleic acid amplification test (CBNAAT) study, and tuberculosis (TB) culture is also done in joint fluid. It can be bedside procedure. Fluid should be sent immediately for culture.

Q7. What are the imaging modalities for septic arthritis?

- *Plain radiograph*: In initial days it may show displacement of soft tissues, edema of soft tissues, and obliteration of normal fat lines. In hip joint arthritis, X-ray may show medial displacement of obturator muscle into the pelvis, lateral displacement or obliteration of the gluteal fat lines, and elevation of Shenton's line with a widened arc.
- *Ultrasound*: In ultrasound of joint, joint effusion, subperiosteal elevation, and fluid collection can be seen. Ultrasound-guided hip aspiration can be done.

	Septic arthritis	Rheumatic fever/ reactive arthritis	Rheumatoid arthritis
CLOG	Large and rapid	Small and absent	Large
CLOG appearance	Curdled milk like	Tight, rope like	Small friable mass
White blood cells	>50,000	15,000–18,000	15,000 around
Glucose (joint fluid/blood × 100%)	30%	75%	75%

- *MRI/CT scan of joint*: MRI is particularly helpful in defining the extension of joint involvement and associated bone involvement. MR imaging is the imaging study of choice and shoud be offered up front. MR imaging gives better spatial resolution than bone scan and is preferred if a surgical procedure to diagnose or drain an abscess is necessary.
- *Radionuclide scan*: It may detect joint involvement very early. It is useful for evaluating sacroiliac joint involvement.

Q8. What is the differential diagnosis?

It depends on the involved joint/joints and the age of the child. For multiple joint involvement, differential diagnosis includes various autoinflammatory disorders like inflammatory bowel disease and rheumatoid conditions.

For hip joint-Perthes disease, toxic synovitis of hip, slipped capital femoral epiphysis, adjacent structures diseases like pyomyositis of muscle, sacroiliitis, and vertebral osteomyelitis are differential diagnosis. Hematological diseases like sickle cell disease, hemophilia, and leukemia can present as acute arthritis. Villonodular synovitis is another diagnosis.

Reactive arthritis due to viral, gastrointestinal or urinary tract infection can resemble septic arthritis.

Q9. What is the treatment?

Treatment is planned as supportive and specific treatment. Supportive treatment includes rest of joint, pain killer, and antipyretic. Some time drainage of pus is needed. Specific antibiotic choice is decided depending upon isolated organism and resistance pattern.

In neonates, antistaphylococcal antibiotics like cloxacillin and broad spectrum cephalosporin-cefotaxime (150–225 mg/kg/day q8h) or cefuroxime (100 mg/kg/day q12h) is recommended. Specific antibiotic can be decided after culture report.

In neonates, possibility of nosocomial infection is suspected and *pseudomonas*, fungi, and MRSA or *Enterobacteriaceae* coverage is advised. In case of MRSA clindamycin (40 mg/kg/day q8h) and vancomycin (15 mg/kg/dose q6h) are alternative when treating community-associated MRSA

(CA-MRSA). In immunocompromised host combination therapy is initiated. Vancomycin and ceftazidime or extended spectrum penicillins and beta-lactam inhibitors and aminoglycoside are recommended.

Duration of antibiotic is individualized depending on age and organism isolated. For *Streptococci, Pneumococci,* and *K. kingae,* 10–14 days treatment is adequate. Longer therapy is recommended for gram-negative organisms and *S. aureus* organism. Normalization of ESR and CRP with improving clinical features will guide for duration of therapy. Oral therapy can be used once patient is afebrile for 3 or 4 days and clinically improving. Cefuroxime can be used orally.

Q10. When surgical intervention is recommended?

Usually hip joint and shoulder joint septic arthritis is considered an emergency because of its vulnerability to cause damage. In other joints, depending upon the severity, aspiration is needed.

Q11. Do we need follow-up of these patients?

Yes, we need follow-up X-ray to check for associated osteomyelitis and regression of soft tissue shadows. Inflammatory parameters (ESR and CRP) are also checked. This is done usually after 3 or 4 weeks of treatment. Long-term complications like joint movement and bone growth need to be checked.

FURTHER READING

1. Greene WB. Osteomyelitis. In: Staheli LT (Ed). Pediatric Orthopedic Secrets. New Delhi: Jaypee Brothers Medical Publishers (P) Ltd.; 1999. pp. 332-7.
2. Kliegmann RM. Nelson Textbook of Pediatrics: First South Asian edition. Amsterdam, Netherlands: Elsevier; 2016. pp. 3322-7.
3. Maraqa NF, Malvarez A. Osteomyelitis. In: Klein JD, Zaoutis TE (Eds). Pediatric Infectious Disease Secrets. Philadelphia: Hanley & Belfus Inc.; 2003. pp. 200-7.

CHAPTER 20

Osteomyelitis

Ketan H Shah

Q1. What is osteomyelitis?

It is inflammation of bone. It could be infectious or noninfectious. It can cause permanent damage to bone or called as death of bone cells. When growth plate is affected it can cause permanent shortening of affected long bones.

Q2. Which are the common organisms causing osteomyelitis?

In neonatal age group the most common organism is *Staphylococcus aureus*. It could be community-associated methicillin-resistant *S. aureus* (CA–MRSA) or hospital-acquired MRSA. *Kingella kingae*, streptococci, *Enterobacteriaceae*, *Pseudomonas*, and *Candida* fungi can also cause osteomyelitis. *Haemophilus influenzae* and pneumococcal bacterial incidence has decreased after vaccination coverage. In neonatal intensive care unit (NICU), fungal infection with sepsis can cause osteomyelitis. In patients having hemoglobinopathy gram-negative bacteria, e.g. *Salmonella* infection is very common. Tuberculosis osteomyelitis is also not uncommon.

Q3. Why *S. aureus* is very common organism?

Staphylococcus aureus has ability to adhere to type one collagen fiber of bone fibrils. It then proliferates and give rise to microcolonies which is surrounded by protective layers, so bacteria is protected from host defenses.

Q4. How the osteomyelitis develops?

It is usually by hematogenous inoculation. Direct inoculation from trauma and spread from adjacent site of infection can occur. The pathogenesis starts with microthrombus formation in sinusoids followed by inoculation of bacteria. Bacteria then proliferate and forms exudates in surrounding areas. These exudates will cause focal necrosis and spread of infection to subperiosteal area.

Q5. What is the difference between acute and chronic osteomyelitis?

Acute osteomyelitis usually presents with high fever and pain. Chronic has slow insidious onset and can have mild symptoms. If disease duration is more than 2 weeks then it is consider as chronic. However, bacterial as well as tuberculosis can be considered in differential diagnosis. Some time etiology may be polymicrobial.

Q6. What are the clinical signs and symptoms of childhood osteomyelitis?
Constitutional signs and symptoms may precede bone symptoms. Fever, malaise, and pain at affected site can occur. Depending upon the affected bone child may have restricted movement of that part. If lower limb is affected, child may present with limping. Pelvic osteomyelitis can present with limp, hip, thigh or abdominal pain. Vertebral osteomyelitis can present as back pain and tenderness. In children, *S. aureus* can present with multiple site involvement. In adjacent area venous thrombosis can develop. This thrombus can cause pulmonary embolism.

Q7. What is Brodie's abscess?
These children will have subacute symptoms and focal findings in metaphyseal area. On X-ray of affected part, radiological lucency and surrounding reactive bone area is seen. This abscess is called Brodie's abscess. The content of abscess is sterile.

Q8. What is unique about neonate and bone infection?
Neonates may have nonspecific symptoms. They may have pseudoparalysis of the affected limb. It may affect multiple bones. Newborn have thin cortex and loose periosteum. This peculiarity increases the risk of spread of infection and destruction of bone structures. It can spread to muscle and soft tissues. In older children, periosteum is thick so spread of infection outside bone is not common. Immature growth plate may rupture in neonates and can cause associated septic arthritis.

- If cephalohematoma is infected osteomyelitis of skull can develop
- After heel puncture (routinely done for blood investigations) calcenum bone osteomyelitis can occur
- Osteitis can be manifestation of syphilis
- Maxillary osteomyelitis is described in newborn
- Hospital-acquired organism can cause serious infection. Gram-negative multidrug-resistant bacteria and fungal infections are common in NICU
- They need long duration of treatment, sometime up to 4–6 weeks.

Q9. Which bones are commonly affected?
Acute hematogenous spread unusually affects long bones. Lower extremity bones are more commonly affected than upper extremity. Nontubular bones including cuboidal and flat bones are less commonly affected. In cuboidal and flat bone calcenum bone is most commonly affected.

Q10. What is the characterization of osteomyelitis in children with hemoglobinopathy?
It occurs in greater frequency in children between 18 and 24 months of age. It affects multiple joints. It is most commonly caused by *Salmonella* species. Staphylococci and other gram-negative organisms can cause osteomyelitis in children. In these children, multiple sites are affected. Sometimes it is difficult to differentiate between bone infarct and osteomyelitis. Bone scan can differentiate between infarction and infection. Multiple episodes of dactylitis and low fever with normal count may favor infarction than infection.

Q11. What are the diagnostic tests for osteomyelitis?
Blood culture before starting antibiotic is important. Bone aspiration or aspiration from adjacent septic joint will help etiological diagnosis. Typically culture is inoculated immediately and kept for more than seven days. *K. kingae* can grow after seven days. Polymerase chain reaction (PCR)-based technology will improve identification of organism.

Leukocytosis, elevated acute phase reactant, erythrocyte sedimentation rate (ESR), and C-reactive protein (CRP) will help in following the progression of the disease. Normal test result does not rule out disease. In initial few days reports may be normal. Cartridge-based nucleic acid amplification test (CBNAAT) study from aspirated material as per need is advised for tuberculosis.

Q12. What is the role of radiology?
Conventional X-rays, ultrasonogram (USG), magnetic resonance imaging (MRI), computer tomography (CT), and bone scan has crucial role to play for establishing diagnosis and for follow-up management. Plain X-ray will look for trauma, suspicious foreign body, and extent of the disease. Soft tissues shadows are displaced in comparison to other side. Lytic changes are not visible unless 40–50% of bone is damaged. Long bones they take 7–10 days for seeing visible damage in X-ray. Radio nucleotide scan will pickup deep lesions and multiple lesions also. MRI of affected part will further define diseased part. MR imaging provides excellent resolution of bone and soft tissue and is useful for visualizing soft tissue abscess associated with osteomyelitis, bone marrow edema, and bone destruction. MRI should be offered upfront and is the modality of choice.

Q13. What is the differential diagnosis?
Hemoglobinopathy like sickle cell disease is important differential diagnosis. The list is long but not restricted. Trauma, fracture, septicemia, septic arthritis, leukemia, lymphoma, bone infraction, thrombophlebitis, histiocytosis, myositis, polymyositis, benign and malignant tumor of bone, vasculitis

phenomena, etc. are important differential diagnosis. Pelvic muscles are most commonly affected in myositis. Limping pain is common manifestation of pelvic muscle myositis or osteomyelitis. MRI will be useful to diagnose polymyositis. Iliopsoas abscess can manifest as limping. Neuroblastoma may be mistaken as bone infection.

Q14. What is chronic recurrent multifocal osteomyelitis (CRMO)?

It is a nonpyogenic, sterile, and inflammatory bone disease considered as autoinflammatory disorder. Family history of autoimmune disorder may be present. Patient may have associated other inflammatory disorders like Crohn's disease, Sweet syndrome, psoriasis, and palmar planter pustulosis.

Chronic recurrent multifocal osteomyelitis has many similarity with SAPHO syndrome (Synovitis, Acne, Pustulosis, Hyperostosis, and Osteitis) and Majeed syndrome (microcytic dyserythropoietic anemia with deficiency of interluekein-1 receptor antagonist and autosomal recessive autoinflammatory disease). CRMO affects bones that are not typical of osteomyelitis like spine, pelvis, clavicle, mandible, and calcenum. It is multifocal and recurrent. MRI and bone scan of whole body study will reveal multifocal bone disease. Usual age of onset is 10 years. Nonsteroidal anti-inflammatory drug (NSAID) and sometime steroid remains main treatment.

Q15. What is the treatment of osteomyelitis?

Antibiotics

Initial choice depends on age and likely pathogen. Empirical antibiotic should cover *S. aureus* and streptococcal bacteria. In NICU and hospital-acquired infection, gram-negative bacteria and fungal infection needs consideration. If MRSA infection is suspected or diagnosed, antibiotic of choice will be vancomycin. Depending upon Gram stain and culture yield antibiotics can be changed.

Empirical choice would be nafcillin or oxacillin [150–200 mg/kg/day q6h intravenous (IV)] and broad spectrum cephalosporin like cefotaxime (150–225 mg/kg/day q8h IV). Cloxacillin/flucloxacillin injections are available in India so it can be used. Vancomycin is recommended for severely ill, bacteremic patient with high chances of MRSA (60 mg/kg/day q8h IV). If child is not severely ill and clindamycin resistance is less than 10% amongst community acquired *S. aureus* organism, clindamycin can be choice of antibiotic (40 mg/kg/day q8h). In penetrating wound injury with osteomyelitis clindamycin remains the choice. Clindamycin has broad spectrum anaerobic activity. Cefazolin (100 mg/kg/day q8h IV) can be used for MRSA and not severely ill patient. For *Streptococci* and *Salmonella* infection, cefotaxime or ceftriaxone can be used. In immune-compromised patient, broad spectrum coverage with vancomycin and ceftazidime or piperacillin-tazobactam and aminoglycoside are recommended. *K. kingae* organism responds to beta-lactam antibiotics.

Duration of therapy

It is individualized depending upon the patient and response. Usual duration is not shorter than 3–4 weeks for *S. aureus*. For *Streptococci, H. influenzae* and *K. Kingae* it may shorter but not less than 2 weeks. ESR, CRP, and clinical condition of patient will guide for further duration of therapy. In immune-compromised patient and for fungal infections duration of treatment is much longer. Oral therapy can be considered if patients' condition improves. Cephalexin, cefuroxime, and clindamycin can be used orally for susceptible bacteria.

Q16. What is the role of surgical therapy?

For frank pus, retained foreign body and for penetrating wound, surgical intervention is recommended. Physical therapy has important role. Passive extension of affected limb and physiotherapy are part of the treatment.

Q17. How to follow-up the patient?

After appropriate antibiotics clinical improvement is seen within 2–3 days. CRP will reduce after 3–4 days. ESR will initially increase for 7–10 days and then fall after 10–14 days. If there is no improvement in 3–4 days, change of antibiotic or revision of diagnosis is needed. Follow-up for range of movement at joint and bone length measurement is important.

FURTHER READING

1. Greene WB. Osteomyelitis. In: Staheli LT (Ed). Pediatric Orthopedic Secrets, 1st edition. New Delhi: Jaypee Brothers Medical Publisher (P) Ltd.; 1999. pp. 332-7.
2. Kapalan SL. Osteomyelitis. In: Klingeman R, Stanton BF, St Geme JW, Schor NF (Eds). Nelson Textbook of Pediatrics: First South Asian Edition. India: Elsevier India; 2016. pp. 3322-7.
3. Maraqa NF, Alvarez AM. Osteomyelitis. In: Klein JD, Zaoutis TE (Eds). Pediatric Infectious Disease Secrets. Philadelphia: Hanley & Belfus, Inc.; 2003. pp. 200-7.

CHAPTER 21

Acute Bacterial Meningitis

Ritabrata Kundu, Aniruddha Ghosh

Q1. When do you suspect acute bacterial meningitis?

Acute bacterial meningitis (ABM) should be suspected in children who look very sick/toxic and present with nonspecific signs of infection like fever, tachycardia, etc. along with one or more of the symptoms and/or signs below:

- Altered sensorium/unconsciousness
- Headache ± Photophobia ± Projectile vomiting
- Neck stiffness
- Septic shock
- Bulging fontanelle
- Kernig's sign
- Brudzinski's sign
- Focal neuro-deficit including seizures, cranial nerve palsies and paresis limbs.

Newborn and young infants may not have a florid clinical picture and just might present with only poor feeding or refusal to feed, lethargy, excessive sleepiness, irritability or inconsolable cry and subtle seizures. So, in every case of neonatal sepsis, index of suspicion should be very high to exclude any possibility of ABM.

Q2. What investigation you would carry out to confirm your diagnosis?

Diagnosis of ABM is confirmed by a timely lumbar puncture and study of the cerebrospinal fluid (CSF). Confirmation of microbial diagnosis depends on Gram stain and culture of CSF.

Raised total leukocyte count in blood with neutrophilic predominance, raised serum markers of sepsis [erythrocyte sedimentation rate (ESR), c-reactive protein (CRP), procalcitonin, etc.], positive blood culture, serological tests of CSF [latex agglutination, polymerase chain reaction (PCR) etc.], neuroimaging studies [computed tomography (CT) scan, magnetic resonance imaging (MRI) scan, etc.] are all supportive investigations.

Q3. What are the contraindications of lumbar puncture (LP)?

Consider deferring lumbar puncture in patients who has:

- *Features of impending cerebral herniation*: Papilledema, pupillary asymmetry, impaired papillary light reflex, abnormal breathing pattern, bradycardia, hypertension or abnormal posturing
- A Glasgow coma scale (GCS) of less than 8 or below or a deteriorating GCS
- Focal neuro deficits
- Repeated convulsions
- Unstable hemodynamics like in shock
- CT or MRI features suggesting blocked CSF drainage (by blood, pus, tumor or coning)
- A local midline septic focus like cellulitis or abscess in the lower back
- Bleeding tendencies like in impairment of coagulation profile.

Q4. How do you interpret a lumbar puncture in a patient who has already received antibiotic and has traumatic LP?

It is very difficult to interpret a CSF report of patient who already received parenteral antibiotic as Gram stain and culture reports are often negative. Cell counts may also fall due to decrease in inflammation. Biochemical markers like CSF glucose, protein, etc. might still give some clues as they are relatively unaltered. In these, multiplex PCR is an upcoming promising method to detect ABM.

It's better to repeat LP if the first LP is traumatic. Biochemical parameters of CSF may alter excepting glucose but Gram stain and cultures also yield good results.

Q5. What is the differential diagnosis of ABM? How LP helps to confirm the diagnosis?

Differentials to be considered are:

- Viral meningitis and encephalitis
- Tubercular meningitis
- Cerebral malaria
- Complex febrile seizures
- Stroke with fever
- Brain abscess.

Lymphocytic predominance with normal sugar levels and negative culture → *Viral meningoencephalitis* (Exceptions: some cases of mumps encephalitis and Japanese encephalitis).

Lymphocytic preponderance with slightly low sugar, high protein and negative culture → *TB meningitis.*

Endemicity, splenomegaly, lack of signs of meningeal irritation, identification of parasite from peripheral blood smears, almost normal CSF studies → *Cerebral malaria.*

Nontoxic look, normal or mildly altered sensorium which recovers quickly, normal CSF studies → *Complex febrile seizures.*

Focal features, papilledema, mildly raised or normal leukocyte count with normal glucose and protein in CSF → *Brain abscess.*

Lack of meningeal irritation, well localized neuro deficit from the onset, less toxicity, findings related to etiology, i.e. congenital heart disease, hematological and metabolic disorders, etc. → *Stroke with fever.*

If LP shows marked polymorphonuclear pleocytosis, CSF glucose less than two-thirds of simultaneous serum glucose, raised CSF protein, positive Gram stain and culture, it confirms ABM.

Q6. How do you choose empirical antibiotics in ABM? How long to treat?

Empirical antibiotics (always parenteral) are to be chosen keeping the following points in mind:

- *Age of the patient:* Etiological microorganism changes like (in decreasing order of incidence):
  - *In neonates:* Gram-negative organisms, *Haemophilus influenzae* type B, *Pneumococcus* group B streptococci
  - *Beyond newborn age up to 5 years: Pneumococcus, Haemophilus influenzae* type B, community-acquired *Staphylococcus, Meningococcus,* Gram-negative organisms
  - *Beyond 5 years throughout adolescence:* Meningococci, *Pneumococcus, Staphylococcus.*
- *Coexisting clinical pointers towards possible organism:* In history and examination these pointers should be kept in mind:
  - Nonblanching rash (*Meningococcus*), associated pneumonia (*Pneumococcus*), otitis media (*Pneumococcus/H. Influenzae Type B*), skin and soft tissue infections, i.e. pyoderma, cellulitis, boils, etc. (*Staphylococcus*), history of immunodeficiency disorder (*Pseudomonas* and other uncommon organism).
- *Antibiotics having good penetration to CSF:* Usual empirical antibiotics are:
  - In case of newborns:
    - *Cefotaxime* (200–300 mg/kg/day in 3–4 divided doses) ± *Amikacin* (15 mg/kg/day in one or two divided doses)
    - *Ampicillin* (300 mg/kg/day in four divided doses) plus *Gentamicin* (7.5 mg/kg/day divided into 2–3 doses).

- Beyond newborn age: *Ceftriaxone* (100 mg/kg/day in two divided doses).
- If severe sepsis or septic shock is the presentation and there is clinical decision to start with higher generation of antibiotic: *Meropenem* (120 mg/kg/day in three divided doses) may be used.
- If *Staphylococcus* or resistant *Pneumococcus* is suspected as causative agent then *Vancomycin* (60 mg/kg/day in four divided doses) is added.
- If, *Pseudomonas* is the suspected agent then *Ceftazidime* (150 mg/kg/day in three to four divided doses) can be the empiric antibiotic of choice.

Duration of antibiotic therapy:

- 3 weeks in case of newborns
- 2–3 weeks in case of older children
- Prolonged duration of 4–6 weeks of therapy is indicated for complicated ABM cases like that in cases of ventriculitis, subdural empyema, etc.

Q7. What are the complications? How to prevent them?

Most children make a full recovery but sometimes serious complications might occur:

- Subdural effusion, empyema
- Ventriculitis
- Hydrocephalus
- Cranial nerve palsies (hearing loss, loss of vision)
- Recurrent seizures
- Cerebral palsy
- Vasculitic stroke
- Syndrome of inappropriate ADH secretion (SIADH)
- Problems with memory and concentration, learning disability
- Coordination, movement and balance problems.

Complications can be prevented or minimized by following measures:

- Prompt diagnosis
- Timely and judicious antibiotic therapy
- Treatment of dehydration, dyselectrolytemia, seizures, shock during acute phase
- Proper neuroprotective strategies
- Steroids in suspected *H. Influenzae type B* cases (Dexamethasone has shown to reduce incidence of hearing loss)
- Routine and daily monitoring of vital parameters, intake-output, appearance of any new neurological signs, nutrition

- Bedside ultrasonography (USG) or other brain imaging to diagnose subdural empyema, stroke, hydrocephalus, abscess formation early and management of that specific complication accordingly
- Appropriate rehabilitative therapy.

Q8. Prevention of ABM.

Acute bacterial meningitis can be prevented by:

- Appropriate vaccination against *H. Influenzae type B, Pneumococcus and Meningococcus*
- Chemoprophylaxis (by oral rifampicin 10 mg/kg/dose 12 hourly for 2 days) to all close contacts of a case of meningococcal meningitis.

CHAPTER 22

Brain Abscess

Nupur Ganguly, Suchi Acharya

Q1. What is brain abscess?

It is a focal pyogenic infection of the brain with thick outer wall seen in one or more areas of the brain. Mostly they are pyogenic in nature and often have a polymicrobial etiology. It is seen mostly in children between 4 and 8 years and neonates and is a neurological emergency. Early diagnosis, judicious use of parenteral antibiotic, and aggressive neurosurgical intervention can reduce the morbidity and mortality.

Q2. What is the incidence of brain abscess in pediatric population?

As compared to general population pediatric population constitute 25–42% of all brain abscesses. As per hospital studies from India there are 8–15 cases per year compared to 1.5 cases reported from USA.

With technological advancement in imaging more cases of brain abscess are being diagnosed leading to apparent increase in the incidence.

Q3. What are the routes of infection in brain abscess?

Contiguous spread: Infection spreads from a nearby site such as sinuses, orofacial region, mastoid, and aural areas and also rarely from meningitis (which is more commonly seen in neonates with citrobacter infection).

Hematogenous spread: Infection spreads through the blood stream like congenital cyanotic heart disease, bacterial endocarditis, arteriovenous malformation of pulmonary vascular bed, lung infections, and skin and abdominal infections.

Direct spread: Penetrating head injuries can lead to retention of bone fragments which serves as a source of infection giving rise to brain abscess. Ocular injuries with sharp penetrating objects can also cause an abscess.

Brain abscesses occurring from contiguous spread are usually single, whereas hematogenous spread are mostly multiple.

Q4. What are the risk factors for development of a brain abscess?

Congenital cyanotic heart disease (most common risk factor) followed by, otitis media, sinusitis, dermal sinus tract, meningitis, shunt infections, diabetes, and immunosuppression.

Q5. What is the pathogenesis of a brain abscess?

Brain is a sanctuary area inherently resistant to infection. Blood brain barrier inhibits the entry of the pathogens, causing less chance of brain abscess following bacteremia commonly seen in infants and children.

Breach in the integrity of the blood brain barrier leads to the influx of the pathogen in the devitalized area or area with poor microcirculation leads to formation of brain abscess.

Brain abscess evolves in four stages and different zones:

Stage 1: Early cerebritis (day 1–3): Characterized by necrotic tissue, local inflammatory response, and marked edema. In this stage there is no demarcation between the lesion and surrounding brain.

Stage 2: Late cerebritis (day 4–10): Characterized by predominant macrophage and lymphocyte infiltrate.

Stage 3: Early encapsulation (day 10–14): Formation of a well-vascularized wall, which is crucial for localizing the lesion and limiting the spread of infection.

Stage 4: Late capsule stage (>day 14) (mature abscess): After 3–4 weeks, the abscess wall gets thickened and facilitates easy excision. It also helps to sequestrate the lesion and protects the surrounding brain tissue.

Various zones are:

- A necrotic center at the innermost part, surrounded by a zone of inflammatory cells and dense collagenous capsule, followed by a layer of neovascularization. All this gives rise to reactive astrocytosis, gliosis, and cerebral edema outside the capsular layer, enhancing the plane of cleavage between the abscess wall and the surrounding tissue.

Q6. Which organisms cause brain abscess?

Agent	***Frequency (%)***
Aerobic and anaerobic streptococci, *Streptococcus melleri*	60–70
Gram-negative aerobic bacilli	20–40
Staphylococcus aureus	10–15
Fungi	10–15
Streptococcus pneumoniae	<1
Haemophilus influenzae, Pseudomonas	<1
Protozoa and helminths (vary geographically)	<1

Q7. What are the usual microbial isolates according to the predisposing condition?

Predisposing conditions	*Microorganisms*
Otitis media, sinusitis, mastoiditis	Streptococci (anaerobic or aerobic), *Bacteroides* and *Prevotella* species, *Enterobacteriaceae*, *S. aureus*, Hib
Dental sepsis	*Fusobacterium*, streptococci, *Prevotella* and *Bacteroides* species
Penetrating trauma	*S. aureus*, streptococci
Lung and pleural infections	*S. aureus*, *Fusobacterium*, *Actinomyces*, *Prevotella* species, streptococci, *Nocardia*
Bacterial endocarditis	*S. aureus*, streptococci
Congenital cyanotic heart disease	Streptococci, *Haemophilus* species, *Bacteroides*
Febrile neutropenia	Gram-negative bacilli, *Aspergillus*, *Candida* species
Transplantation	*Aspergillus* species, *Candida* species, *Mucorales*, *Enterobacteriaceae*, *Nocardia* species, *Toxoplasma gondii*
HIV infection	*Toxoplasma gondii*, *Nocardia* species, *Mycobacterium* species, *Cryptococcus neoformans*

(Hib: *Haemophilus influenzae* type b; HIV: human immunodeficiency virus)

Q8. What are the signs and symptoms of a brain abscess?

Symptoms are varied. In younger children they are nonspecific like irritability, excessive cry, poor feeding, and vomiting. Can also present with fever, bulged fontanelle, and convulsion.

Older children can present with headache, fever, vomiting, behavioral abnormalities, gait abnormalities, and convulsion. They may have focal neurodeficit manifestations like hemiparesis, dysphasia, ataxia, and nystagmus.

Q9. How is a brain abscess diagnosed?

The diagnosis of a brain abscess is made clinically by specific signs and symptoms and applying diagnostic testing. The diagnostic tests are as follows:

Blood tests: Presence of nonspecific biochemical markers of infection such as moderate leukocytosis and raised C-reactive protein (CRP). Blood culture often sterile unless there is hematogenous spread. Other lab investigations remain unremarkable.

Neuroimaging: Magnetic resonance imaging (MRI) with gadolinium enhancement has now become the investigation of choice. It is more sensitive for detecting early cerebritis, necrosis, and edema. It is also the most sensitive tool for detecting posterior fossa and brain stem abscess. On MRI cerebritis appear as hypointensity on T1-weighted images and hyperintensity in T2-weighted images **(Figs. 1A and B)**.

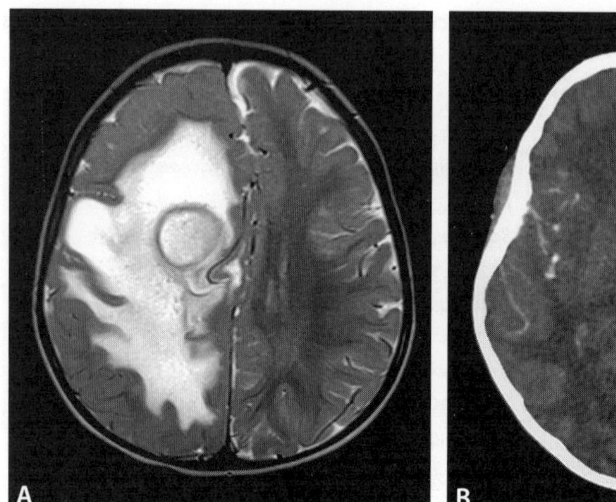

Figs. 1A and B: (A) Contrast MRI brain showing abscess with extensive edema in right frontoparietal lobe causing mass effect and midline shift; (B) MRI brain showing multiple brain abscess 2–3 cm in size in left frontal lobe with perifocal edema and mass effect. (MRI: magnetic resonance imaging)

Newer modalities of MRI such as diffusion-weighted imaging (DWI) and susceptibility-weighted imaging (SWI) can further differentiate between brain abscess and necrotic tumors.

Computed tomography (CT) scan helps in detection of site number and location of abscess. It is readily available and can be used for monitoring the progression of the disease after initiation of therapy. Stereotactic CT-guided aspiration of abscess and biopsy. The aspirate should be sent for bacterial, mycobacterial and fungal stain, culture, and nucleic acid amplification testing (NAAT).

High resolution cranial ultrasonography: It can help in the diagnosis of brain abscess and subdural empyema through open anterior fontanel in neonates.

Lumbar puncture: It is contraindicated in brain abscess due to mass effect and risk of herniation. If done, may have normal cerebrospinal fluid (CSF) findings unless the abscess has ruptured into the ventricular system. If ventriculitis sets in following rupture of the brain abscess there is marked leukocytosis, elevated protein, hypoglycorrhachia, and elevated lactate.

Q10. What is the treatment for a brain abscess?

Brain abscess is a medical emergency and needs immediate hospitalization. Initiation of empiric antibiotic therapy is to be started upfront with close monitoring. Draining of abscess and/or surgical excision is to be done when needed. Empirical antibiotics should be changed as per the culture sensitivity [minimum inhibitory concentrations (MICs)], central nervous system (CNS) penetration of antibiotics and its activity in the abscess cavity.

Symptomatic treatment should be given to control seizures, fever, and/or other conditions that may be present.

As such no guideline is available for the exact duration of antibiotic treatment for brain abscess. But usually 6–8 weeks is recommended, however after surgical excision, a shorter course of 4–6 weeks may be sufficient.

Q11. Which empirical antibiotics are given in brain abscess?

To cover the most common organisms of brain abscess, empirical antibiotics of choice vancomycin, third-generation cephalosporin, and metronidazole. In case of cyanotic congenital heart disease, ampicillin-sulbactam is to be added apart from third-generation cephalosporin and metronidazole. In case of suspected gram-negative infection and anaerobes, the choice of antibiotic is meropenem.

Infected ventriculoperitoneal (VP) shunt giving rise to abscess, the choice is vancomycin and ceftazidime. In neonates infected with *Citrobacter*, third-generation cephalosporin and aminoglycoside are used. In case of suspected *Listeria monocytogenes* infection one can add ampicillin. Antifungal like amphotericin B is to be added in immunocompromised patients along with broad spectrum antibiotics.

Q12. What are the conditions where only medical management is indicated in a brain abscess?

Medical management is to be continued in case of multiple abscesses, small size abscess less than 2.5 cm, if any concomitant meningitis, ependymitis, and in early cerebritis stage who is improving with antibiotics.

Q13. What are the surgical therapies available for brain abscess?

Stereotactic-guided aspiration and excision of brain abscess are the surgical modalities of choice.

Q14. What are the indications for aspiration of brain abscess?

When the abscess is encapsulated, causing mass effect leading to increased intracranial tension.

Q15. What are the indications for excision of brain abscess?

Traumatic abscess (contain foreign body and bone fragment), fungal abscess, gas-containing abscess, large (>2.5 cm), multiloculated, and posterior fossa abscess are the indications for surgical excision of brain abscess.

Q16. What is the role of corticosteroid in brain abscess?

It is indicated when there is profound cerebral edema, herniation, and ventriculitis or rupture of abscess into ventricles.

Q17. What are the poor prognostic markers for brain abscess?

Poor prognostic markers of brain abscess are delayed or missed diagnosis, inappropriate antibiotics, multiple, deep, or multiloculated abscesses, ventricular rupture (80–100% mortality), fungal or any resistant pathogens, neurological compromise at presentation, rapidly progressive neuroimpairment, immunosuppressed host, and poor localization, especially in the posterior fossa.

Q18. What are the long-term morbidities of a brain abscess?

These are seizure, focal neurodeficit (hemiparesis and cranial nerve abnormalities), cognitive dysfunction, and hydrocephalus.

FURTHER READING

1. Brouwer MC, Tunkel AR, McKhann GM, et al. Brain abscess. N Engl J Med. 2014;371:447-56.
2. Prober CG, Mathew R. Brain abscess. In: Kliegman RM, St Geme J, Schor NF (Eds). Nelson Textbook of Pediatrics, 20th edition. Philadelphia: Elsevier; 2016. pp. 2949-50.
3. Saez-Llorens X, Guevara JN. Parameningeal infections. In: Cherry J, Harrison G, Kaplan S, Steinbach W, Hotez P (Eds). Textbook of Pediatric Infectious Diseases, 8th edition. Philadelphia: Elsevier; 2018. pp. 336-45.
4. Weinberg GA, Thompson-Stone R. Bacterial infections of the nervous system. In: Swaiman KF, Ashwal S, Ferriero DM, Schor NF, Finkel RS, Gropman AL, Pearl PL, Shevell MI (Eds). Pediatric Neurology, 6th edition. Philadelphia: Elsevier; 2018. pp. 883-94.

CHAPTER 23

Ring Lesions

Ritesh Shah

Q1. What are the different causes of ring enhancing lesion on MRI?

Few common causes of ring enhancing lesions are granulomatous lesions [like neurocysticercosis (NCC), tuberculoma], brain abscess, fungal infections, demyelination, metastasis and subacute infarcts.

Q2. How to differentiate NCC from tuberculoma on MRI?

Clinically both can present as single seizure so sometimes we have to differentiate on basis of neuroimaging. Neurocysticercosis are usually small (<20 mm), single or multiple lesions with smooth margin, cystic lesion with less edema, occasional mural nodule and mainly located at gray-white matter junction without associated meningitis most of the times while tuberculoma are larger (>20 mm) single or multiple lesion with irregular margin, solid lesion with severe edema and more commonly located in posterior fossa with associated meningitis many times.

Q3. How to treat NCC?

Neurocysticercosis is treated with anticonvulsants, antiparasitic (cysticidal) and anti-inflammatory (steroids). Appropriate treatment of NCC is matter of debate. There are different views about use of anticonvulsants, cysticidal drugs, and steroids. We will try to present best suggestions based on currently available evidence.

Q4. Should the cysticidal be used and how?

Cysticidal treatment aims to destroy live cysts on the assumption that once inactive they will cause fewer symptoms. Faster resolution of neuroimaging lesion is proven in many studies and beneficial effect in terms of seizure control is reported in some studies. Although albendazole and praziquantel both have been found effective in NCC, albendazole is better tolerated and less expensive. The usual regime of albendazole is 15 mg/kg/day in to two divided doses for 7–28 days. Both short (7 day) and long (28 day) duration therapy found to be equally effective for parenchymal NCC.

Q5. How to go about steroids in NCC?

Steroids are generally given to reduce the perilesional edema. They are started 1-2 days before starting albendazole and continued for next 2–3 days with objective of minimizing any inflammatory response that might be flared up by cysticidal therapy. Usually prednisolone 2 mg/kg/day is used, in children with raised ICT intravenous dexamethasone may be used.

Q6. How to treat tuberculoma?

Tuberculoma is treated with antitubercular treatment (ATT) regime and anti-inflammatory. ATT regime: 2 HRZE (Intensive Phase) + 7 HRE (Continuation phase) Doses: H-Isoniazid (@ 10 mg/kg), R-Rifampicin (@ 10 mg/kg), Z-Pyrazinamide (@ 30–35 mg/kg), E-Ethambutol (@ 20–25 mg/kg).

Q7. How long to treat tuberculoma?

There is lack of evidence to optimum treatment duration in CNS tuberculoma but latest guidelines suggest ATT for 9–12 months with repeat neuroimaging at 3 months and 9–12 months to monitor response to treatment. In few cases maintenance phase needs to be continued for 18–24 months.

Q8. What is the role of steroids in tuberculoma?

Paradoxical reaction with increase in size and number of lesions can occur usually in first 3 months and requires treatment with steroids with ATT. Steroids should be given at the rate 2 mg/kg/day for 4 weeks followed by reducing course over next 4 weeks.

Q9. What is the treatment approach for brain abscess?

Brain abscess is treated with antibiotics, antibiotics + aspiration or surgical excision depending on clinical condition, location of abscess and duration of illness. Early treatment with antibiotics as soon as diagnosis is made. In unknown cases start with combination therapy with vancomycin, 3rd generation cephalosporin and metronidazole. If histories suggestive of any etiology like trauma, congenital heart disease, primary focus like otitis media, mastoditis then choose antibiotics appropriately. In case of immunocompromised host add amphotericin B (antifungal) in addition to broad spectrum antibiotics. Duration of antibiotic therapy depends on organism and response to treatment but usually 4–6 weeks. If lesion is causing mass effect or with raised ICT treat with antibiotics + aspiration.

Q10. When to do surgical excision for brain abscess?

Surgery is indicated when abscess is more than 2.5 cm in diameter, multiloculated lesion, lesion in posterior fossa, gas is present in abscess or fungus is identified.

FURTHER READING

1. Kliegman RM, Stanton B, Geme JS, et al. Brain Abscess. In: Nelson Textbook of Pediatrics, 20th edition. Philadelphia: Elsevier, 2016.
2. Singhi P, Singhi S. Neurocysticercosis in children. Indian J Pediatr. 2009;76(5): 537-45.
3. WHO. Guidance for national tuberculosis programs on management of tuberculosis in children, second edition. Geneva: World Health Organization; 2014.

SECTION 3

Healthcare-associated Infections and Special Situations

CHAPTER 24

Ventilator-associated Pneumonia

Bharat Mehra, Amarjeet Chitkara

Q1. How do you suspect ventilator-associated pneumonia (VAP) in a ventilated child?

Ventilator-associated pneumonia is defined as "new onset of pneumonia in a patient after 48 hours of mechanical ventilation". One has to rely on combination of clinical, microbiological, and radiological criteria. When a child who has been relatively stable on mechanical ventilator develops at least three of the following:

- Fever (>38.0°C or >100.4°F) or hypothermia (<36.0°C or <96.8°F)
- Leukopenia (≤4,000 white blood cell [WBC]/mm^3) or leukocytosis (≥15,000 WBC/mm^3)
- New onset of purulent sputum or change in character of sputum, or increased respiratory secretions, or increased suctioning requirements
- New onset or worsening cough, or dyspnea, apnea, or tachypnea
- Rales or bronchial breath sounds
- Worsening gas exchange [for example, O_2 desaturations (pulse oximetry < 94%), increased oxygen requirements, or increased ventilator demand]

Using the above set of variables, a clinical pulmonary infection score (CPIS) is calculated and this score helps in taking a decision to start antibiotics, as well as monitor a child with diagnosis of VAP.

Q2. Which investigations are helpful in diagnosing VAP?

Apart from total leukocyte count and chest X-ray, microbiological evidence by growing a pathogen from respiratory secretions should be done. Ideally respiratory secretions should be collected with help of flexible fiber optic bronchoscopy and taking bronchoalveolar lavage (BAL). Other methods are blind bronchial sampling (BBS), blind protected sampling brush (BPSB), and taking a tracheal aspirate. Simply obtaining a positive culture is not enough as airways are frequently colonized with organisms. CDC recommends bacterial growth of more than 10^4 CFU/mL in BAL; more than 10^3 CFU/mL in BPSB as the criteria for significant growth.

Q3. What are the common microorganisms implicated in VAP?

Ventilator-associated pneumonia is commonly caused by hospital-acquired gram-negative pathogens such as *Klebsiella, Escherichia coli, Pseudomonas aeruginosa*; gram-negative coccobacilli such *Acinetobacter baumannii*; and methicillin-resistant *Staphylococcus aureus*. Aspiration of oropharyngeal secretions around endotracheal (ET) tube is commonly implicated as the primary route of bacterial entry into trachea. These gram-negative organisms are frequently being identified as multidrug-resistant (MDR) and are result of overzealous and misuse of antibiotics. In immunocompromised patients' fungal pathogens such *Candida* and *Aspergillus* are also seen.

Q4. What should be the empirical therapy for VAP?

The decision for the choice of antimicrobial therapy depends on various risk factors for MDR pathogens as well as local microbial prevalence and antibiogram. These are:

- Recent antimicrobial therapy for more than 7 days within the past 30–90 days
- Hospitalization more than or equal to 5 days, recent hospitalization (at least 2 days in past month)
- Structural lung disease
- Systemic corticosteroid therapy (>10 mg prednisolone equivalent daily) and immunosuppressive disease or medications
- Chronic dialysis
- Resident in chronic care facility
- Home infusion or wound care
- Known exposure to resistant pathogen (household or community)
- Malnutrition.

In the presence of above risk factors, there is high likelihood for MDR pathogens and warrant combination therapy.

- Piperacillin-tazobactam or meropenem or imipenem ± aminoglycoside
- In intensive care units (ICUs) where MRSA prevalence is high, vancomycin could be added empirically.

Importantly, once a pathogen is identified, de-escalation to monotherapy appears to be safe and preferred, provided there is clinical improvement.

Q5. What should be the duration of antimicrobial therapy?

Decision of antimicrobial therapy is based on clinical progress of child and the organism grown. Clinical response can be monitored by improvement in modified clinical pulmonary infection score (mCPIS) score and radiological improvement. If there is good clinical response, absence of risk factors for MDR pathogens and absence of any positive culture then antibiotics can be stopped by 7 days. However, if any of the above criteria is not satisfied then antibiotics should be continued for 14–21 days.

Q6. How can I decrease the incidence of VAP in my hospital/unit?

Ventilator-associated pneumonia bundles are a series of evidence-based measures which implemented together have shown to decrease the incidence of VAP. Implementing these bundles should be the standard of care in each unit. These are:

- Head end elevation 30–45° for intubated/sick patients
- Regular oral care with chlorhexidine 0.12%
- Clearing of oral secretions followed by ET secretions while suctioning
- Avoid gastric overdistension
- Avoid unplanned extubation and reintubation
- Use of cuffed ET tube (where feasible) and maintain adequate cuff pressures
- Change of ventilator circuits when visibly soiled or malfunctioning
- Implementation of protocol to reduce sedation and minimize the duration of mechanical ventilation
- Reduce the length of treatment for VAP except for nonfermenting gram-negative bacilli.

CHAPTER 25

Central Line-associated Bloodstream Infection

Narayanappa D

Q1. What is included in the definition of a central line (CL)?

A CL for purposes of surveillance for central line-associated bloodstream infection (CLABSI) is defined as a vascular infusion device that terminates at or close to the heart or in one of the great vessels. The following are considered great vessels for the purpose of reporting CL infections and counting CL days in the National Healthcare Safety Network (NHSN) system: Aorta, pulmonary artery, superior vena cava, inferior vena cava, brachiocephalic veins, internal jugular veins, subclavian veins, external iliac veins, and common femoral veins.

Q2. What are the types of central venous catheters (CVCs)?

There are several types of CVCs:

- Non-tunneled CVC: Most common type
- A peripherally inserted central catheter (PICC) line is placed into a vein in the arm. Used in neonates most often for parenteral nutrition.
- A tunneled catheter is surgically placed into a vein in the chest or neck and then passed under the skin. One end of the catheter comes out through the skin so medicines can be given right into the catheter. Used for long-term use, chemotherapy, and blood transfusion in thalassemia. Has less risk of CLABSI.
- An implanted port is similar to a tunneled catheter, but an implanted port is placed entirely under the skin. Medicines are given by a needle placed through the skin into the catheter. An implanted port is not as visible as a tunneled catheter, does not require as much daily care, and does not get in the way of a patient's regular activities as much as a PICC line or a tunneled catheter might.
- Umbilical arterial catheter (UAC) and umbilical venous catheter (UVC)—umbilical lines in neonates.

Q3. What is CLABSI rate?

Central line-associated bloodstream infection is most common healthcare-associated infection in pediatric age group. Although data are sparse, in one study CLABSI rates were:

- 5.7 per 1,000 catheter-days in four inpatient wards
- 5.2 per 1,000 catheter-days for medical.

National Healthcare Safety Network CLABSI Rates

From 2006–2008 NHSN report, pooled mean CLABSI rates were:

- Medical surgical intensive care units (ICUs) = 1.5–2.1 per 1,000 catheter-days
- Medical surgical wards = 1.2 per 1,000 catheter-days
- In hemodialysis = 1–4 per 1,000 catheter-days.

Q4. How to calculate CLABSI rate?

CLABSI rate is calculated per 1000 central line days by dividing the number of CLABSIs identified by the number of central line days and multiplying the result by 1000 over a given period of time

CLABSI RATE = CLABSIs identified/Central line days *1,000

How to calculate central line days is , ideally, at the same time each day, count the number of patients with one or more temporary CLs. At the end of the month sum up these counts and use as a denominator for calculating CLABSI rates. At the end of the month see that the completed form is forwarded to the infection control professional (ICP) at your hospital. The ICP will use this to calculate a CLABSI rate. This gives us the central line days per the month and counting the number of new CLABSIs identified in the given month , CLABSI rate for the month can be calculated.

Please note: If a patient has more than one CL on a given day, this is counted only as one CL day.

If a CL is being routinely flushed to keep it from clotting; no other infusions or withdrawals are done through the line, this contributes one CL day to the monthly total for each day this is in place.

Q5. How to calculate CL days?

Ideally, at the same time each day, count the number of patients with one or more temporary CLs. At the end of the month sum up these counts and use as a denominator for calculating CLABSI rates. At the end of the month see that the completed form is forwarded to the infection control professional (ICP) at your hospital. The ICP will use this to calculate a CLABSI rate.

Please note:

- If a patient has *more than one CL on a given day,* this is counted only as one CL day.

- If a CL is being routinely flushed to keep it from clotting; no other infusions or withdrawals are done through the line, this contributes one CL day to the monthly total for each day this is in place.

Q6. What is device utilization (DU) ratio?

Device utilization (DU) ratio, i.e. Central line DU Ratio = central line days/ patient days .

Central line days are calculated by the above mentioned method.

Patient days are the total number of days that patients are in the ICU over the given duration of time for which rate is being calculated. It is to be calculated in a similar way , at same time each day , count the total number of patients in ICU and sum up these counts over given time frame.

The DU ratio measures the proportion of total patient days in which CLs were used.

Q7. What is difference between colonization and CLABSI?

Colonization: Presence of microorganisms on skin, mucous membranes, etc. which are not causing adverse clinical signs or symptoms.

Q8. What is CLABSI?

Centers for Disease Control and Prevention (CDC) defines CLABSI as primary bloodstream infection (BSI) in a patient who had a CL at least for the last 48 hours period before the development of BSI and is not related to an infection at another site.

Q9. What is the difference between CLABSI and Catheter-related bloodstream infection (CRBSI)?

- A CLABSI is operationally very easy and is a surveillance definition, nonspecific, can lead to over diagnosis.
- A CRBSI is a clinical definition, more specific and slightly complex, removal of catheter not possible most of the times, laboratory inadequacy, and cost are its disadvantages.
- A CLABSI is being used more commonly.

Q10. What is the definition of CRBSI?

A CRBSI definition criterion varies depending on whether catheter is removed or not.

- *If catheter is removed*: 5 cm from its tip should be cultured by roll plate method, growth more than 15 colony forming unit (CFU)/plate or by quantitative broth culture, more than 10^2 CFU/mL and same organism also grown from peripheral venipuncture site for growth to be significant, else considered as colonization.

- *If catheter is kept in situ*: Culture should be sent from catheter site as well as peripheral sample (if multilumen catheter—send from all lumens)
  Catheter site culture should have colony counts greater than or equal to three times that of peripheral sample. If done by continuous automated monitoring catheter sample should detect growth at least 120 minutes before peripheral sample—differential time to positivity (DTP) criteria.
- *If peripheral sample is unavailable*: Fivefold or more difference between two lumen samples is diagnostic.

Q11. If CL tip culture had more than 15 CFU of *Staphylococcus aureus* but all blood cultures are negative. Is this a CLABSI?
No. This often is a precursor to a BSI but instead this meets NHSN definition of localized infection of the CL insertion site. NHSN classifies this as an infection of the vein. It is fine to include this in the surveillance of infectious complications of CLs. However, do not use this in the calculation of the CLABSI rate. This rate is limited to CL-associated BSIs/total number of CL days × the constant of 1,000 only.

Q12. Is routine culture of catheter tip recommended?
Routinely it is not recommended, should be done only if CLABSI is suspected.

Q13. When to remove CVC and when not to?
Catheter sites should be monitored daily visually through intact dressing or by palpation for tenderness, erythema, swelling, induration or purulence. If any unusual signs, fever without focus or other manifestations suggesting CLABSI, the dressing should be completely removed and site should be examined to decide whether to remove or not.

Q14. How often CL to be replaced?
Central venous catheter to be replaced only if its malfunctioning or suspected to cause CLABSI. Routine replacement of CVCs after 7 days or exchange over a guidewire has not reduced CLABSI and is not recommended. Exchange over a guidewire is acceptable and preferred than using a new site.

Q15. If CL was inserted in the operating room, can we exclude this case from the CLABSI rate because we did not insert it here in our ICU?
No. Even though it was inserted elsewhere, the key factors are that your patient had a CL in for 48 hours or more before onset and was in your ICU. This case should be included in the numerator for the monthly calculation of this unit's CLABSI rate. If this happens often use additional analysis—perhaps Keystone's investigating a defect tool—to determine if units from which you receive patients are consistently using evidence-based processes

to prevent these infections. If not then collaborate with these areas to improve performance and prevent these infections.

Q16. What is the pathogenesis of CLABSI?
More common mechanisms:

- Pathogen migration along external surface—more common early (< 7 days)
- Hub contamination with intraluminal colonization—more common (>10 days)

Less common mechanisms:

- Hematogenous seeding from another source
- Contaminated infusates
- Certain strains like coagulase-negative staphylococci (CoNS) and *Candida* (especially in presence of glucose) have increased ability to adhere to the catheter and produce a biofilm, made of extracellular polysaccharides, which acts as protective barrier against host defense and antibiotics.

Q17. What are the risk factors of CLABSI?
Modifiable risk factors
Characteristic risk factor hierarchy

1. *Insertion circumstances*: Emergency > elective
2. *Skill of inserter*: General > specialized
3. *Insertion site*: Femoral > subclavian
4. *Skin antisepsis*: 70% alcohol, 10% povidone-iodine > 2% chlorhexidine
5. *Catheter lumens*: Multilumen > single lumen
6. *Duration of catheter use*: Longer duration, greater risk
7. *Barrier precautions*: Submaximal > maximal
8. *Others*: Condition of the patient (immunosuppression, severity of illness), location in the hospital (trauma and surgical units more risk).

Q18. Multilumen catheter has more risk than single lumen?
Evidence shows higher the number of lumens greater the risk of CLABSI.

Q19. Why emergency insertion is associated with more risk than elective?
With emergency insertion aseptic insertion practices cannot be followed strictly.

Q20. Does type of infusate has role in increased risk?
Yes, infusion of lipids is associated with CoNS and *Candida* infections, especially in very low birth weight infants.

Q21. Which organisms are more commonly associated with CLABSI?
According to National Nosocomial Infections Surveillance (NNIS) data (1992–1999), CONS (37%), S. aureus (13%), Enterococcus (13%), gram-negative bacilli (14%), Candida (8%) are the most commonly involved organisms.

Indian data: Overall profile is same but gram-negatives are much more common than CONS.

Q22. What is the proper insertion practice of a CL?
Insertion bundle is to be utilized:

- Chlorhexidine for skin antisepsis
- Maximal sterile barrier precautions [e.g. mask, cap (i.e. similar to those worn in the operation theatre), gown, sterile gloves, and large sterile drape]
- Hand hygiene
- "Bundling" all needed supplies in one area (e.g. a cart or a kit) helps ensure items are available for use
- Consider using NHSN central line insertion practices (CLIP) option.

Q23. What is the role of catheter material?
Polyvinyl or polyethylene catheters are associated with higher infection rates.

Q24. What are the preferred agents for skin cleansing?

- Chlorhexidine is the preferred agent for skin cleansing for both CL insertion and maintenance.
- Tincture of iodine, an iodophor, and 70% alcohol are alternatives.

  Recommended application methods and contact time should be followed for maximal effect. Prior to use should ensure agent is compatible with catheter:
- Alcohol may interact with some polyurethane catheters.
- Some iodine-based compounds may interact with silicone catheters.

Q25. What is the recommendation for prophylactic topical antibiotic at insertion site?
Use of povidone-iodine ointment at insertion site reduced colonization in many studies and is recommended. However, due to emergence of resistance, increased colonization with *Candida*, they are not used prophylactically.

Q26. Traditional versus transparent dressings, which is better?
Transparent polyurethane dressings: Direct inspection, needs to be changed less often, changed every 7th day.

Traditional gauze dressings: Changed every 2nd day.

Q27. What is the appropriate agent for cleansing hubs?
70% alcohol.

Q28. What is the use of antibiotic lock?
This involves leaving a supraphysiologic dose of antibiotic solution in the hub, most commonly used is vancomycin, which has shown to be effective in multiple studies.

Q29. What is the preferred site of insertion?
- Subclavian route least infection rate but high risk of mechanical complications, pneumothorax, and difficult to stop bleeding.
- In patients with renal failure, subclavian site should be avoided as it might lead to stenosis, mainly future fistula development difficult.
- Femoral site should be avoided due to an increased risk of infection and deep venous thrombosis.
- No difference in CLABSI rates in femoral versus nonfemoral routes according to many pediatric studies.
- No site is preferable over other, matter of personal preference.

Q30. What are antimicrobial impregnated catheters?
- Two types with most supporting evidence: Minocycline-rifampin and chlorhexidine-silver sulfadiazine.
- Platinum-silver catheter available but less evidence to support use.
- These may be appropriate for patients whose catheter is expected to be used for more than 5 days.

Q31. What are the considerations for arterial lines?
Infection rate is lower than CVCs, but arterial lines should be removed as soon as possible. Radial, dorsalis pedis, and posterior tibial are used. Brachial artery should not be used. Femoral or axillary artery can also be used not are not preferred.

Q32. What are the considerations for umbilical lines?
Both are associated with similar CLABSI rates, full barrier precaution may be maintained. While using UAC monitoring of lower limbs for signs of vascular insufficiency should be done, if present catheter must be removed. Low dose heparin (0.25–1 IU/mL) should be added to infused fluid to avoid thrombotic complications. UAC can be used for not more than 5 days and UVC till 14 days.

Q33. How do you manage CLABSI?
Suspected CLABSI with septic shock, local infection or metastatic complications:

- Send cultures
- Remove catheter
- Start empirical antibiotic therapy.

Q34. What is the antibiotic policy for CLABSI?

Choice of antibiotic depends on:

- Severity of illness
- Local ICU patterns
- Prior antibiotic use.

Empiric therapy in CRBSI (pending culture report):

- For gram-negative activity:
  - β-lactam/β-lactamase inhibitors—piperacillin-tazobactam (100 mg/kg/dose TID) (or)
  - Carbapenems-meropenem (40–60 mg/kg TID)/fourth-generation cephalosporins for severe cases
  - Colistin (50,000 IU/kg/day TID) if carbapenem already in use or resistance noticed based on local antibiogram in ICU.
- Gram-positive activity:
  - Vancomycin (60 mg/kg/day QID)
  - Cloxacillin (if MRSA is rare in hospital—to cover—CoNS)
- Critically ill patients: Add aminoglycoside.

After culture report: If

- CoNS (most common, least virulent, and with less sepsis)
  - Cloxacillin—drug of choice in MSSA
  - Vancomycin/teicoplanin/daptomycin if MRSA
  - If catheter removed 5–7 days therapy will suffice
  - If retained, 10–14 days therapy after a negative blood culture is attained
- *S. aureus*:
  - More virulent whether it is MSSA or MRSA
  - Serious risk of systemic infection and endocarditis
  - Catheter to be removed
  - If MSSA—cloxacillin and if MRSA—vancomycin
  - Usual duration—14 days
  - If systemic complications like endocarditis or immunocompromised patients
  - Catheter in situ treat for 4–6 weeks
- Gram-negative bacilli:
  - Remove CVC
  - Beta-lactam antibiotic, if sensitive is first choice (as cephalosporins are being resistant)

- Resistant to beta-lactam—meropenem or colistin preferred
- 10–14 days
- *Candida*:
  - Remove CVC
  - Fluconazole—initial choice for 14 days
  - If patient received azoles last 3 months, echinocandin like caspofungin can be used.

Q35. How to treat CLABSI with multilumen catheter?

Antibiotic should be rotated through different lumens unless the infected lumen is identified.

Q36. Which is the most common organism involved in CLABSI?

CoNS, most common, least virulent, and with less sepsis

- Cloxacillin—drug of choice in MSSA
- Vancomycin/teicoplanin/daptomycin if MRSA
- If catheter removed 5–7 days therapy will suffice
- If retained, 10–14 days therapy after a negative blood culture is attained.

Q37. Which is the most virulent organism involved?

Staphylococcus aureus:

- Catheter to be removed
- If MSSA—cloxacillin and if MRSA—vancomycin
- Usual duration—14 days.

Q38. Decision making on removal of catheter.

- Safest option is to remove the catheter for culture, but if another access is very difficult, CL is crucial for ongoing management.
- Long-term lines in stable patients, antibiotics are always tried with catheter in situ and up to 75–90% of catheters could be salvaged.
- Catheter can be kept in situ in a stable patient than in a patient with severe sepsis and any clinical deterioration should prompt removal.
- Daily culture to be sent (paired i.e. catheter and peripheral sample) and if culture is positive 72 hours after starting antibiotics then also catheter is removed.

Q39. What is the ideal duration of therapy?

Ideally repeat culture to be sent even if catheter is removed and duration is to be counted from the day of first positive culture. Usual duration is 10–14 days for *S. aureus*, catheter is be removed and 4–6 weeks of antibiotic is recommended, if catheter is kept in situ, culture is positive after 72 hours in immunosuppressed, diabetics patients with other intravascular prosthetic devices.

Q40. How to prevent CLABSI?

- Interventions:
  - Promotion of best practices
    - Maximal barrier precautions
    - Use of chlorhexidine for skin cleansing prior to insertion
    - Avoidance of femoral site for CL
    - Use of recommended insertion site dressing practices
  - Removal of CL when no longer needed
- Educational module about BSI prevention
- Engagement of leadership and clinicians
- Standard tools for recording adherence to best practices
- Standardizing catheter insertion kits
- Measurement of CLABSI and reporting of rates back to facilities.

Q41. What are the core prevention strategies?

- Removing unnecessary CL
- Following proper insertion practices
- Facilitating proper insertion practices
- Complying with hand hygiene recommendations
- Adequate skin antisepsis
- Choosing proper CL insertion sites
- Performing adequate hub/access port disinfection
- Providing education on CL maintenance and insertion.

Q42. What are the supplemental measures?

- Implementing chlorhexidine bathing
- Using antimicrobial-impregnated catheters
- Applying chlorhexidine site dressings.

Q43. What is chlorhexidine bathing?

Daily bathing with 2% chlorhexidine-impregnated cloths decreased the rate of BSIs.

Q44. What is the role of chlorhexidine dressings?

- Chlorhexidine-impregnated sponge dressings have been shown to decrease rates of CLABSIs in some studies and not in others.
- These dressings may be an option when core interventions have not decreased rates of CLABSI to established goal.

Q45. What are maximal sterile barrier precautions?

- A mask, cap, sterile gown, and sterile gloves are to be worn by all health care personnel involved in the catheter insertion procedure.

- The patient is to be covered with a large (full-body) sterile drape during catheter insertion.

Q46. How to minimize usage of CL?

- In one study, 9% of CLs outside of ICU deemed inappropriate
- Perform daily assessment of the need for the CL and promptly discontinue CLs that are no longer required
- Nursing staff should be encouraged to notify physicians of CLs that are unnecessary
- Use peripheral catheters instead—these generally have lower rates of BSIs than CL.

Q47. What is CLABSI bundle?

This includes elements about proper insertion, maintenance, and monitoring practices of CL. Includes hand hygiene, maximal barrier precautions, chlorhexidine antisepsis, optimal catheter site selection, daily review of line, prompt removal if unnecessary, keeping clean, and secure line intact.

FURTHER READING

1. Bloodstream Infection Event (Central Line-Associated Bloodstream Infection and Non-central Line Associated Bloodstream Infection), CDC January 2019 CDC National and State Healthcare-Associated Infections Progress Report, published October 2018, available at https://www.cdc.gov/hai/data/portal/progress-report.html.
2. CDC. (2002). Guidelines for the Prevention of Intravascular Catheter-Related Infections. [online] Available from https://www.cdc.gov/mmwr/preview/mmwrhtml/rr5110a1.htm?vm=r [Accessed December 2018].
3. CDC. (2016). Central Line-associated Bloodstream Infection (CLABSI). [online] Available from https://www.cdc.gov/hai/bsi/bsi.html [Accessed December 2018].
4. CDC/NHSN Patient Safety Component Manual Summary of Revisions, January 2018.
5. Edwards JR, Peterson KD, Mu Y, et al. National Healthcare Safety Network (NHSN) report: data summary for 2006 through 2008, issued December 2009. Am J Infect Control. 2009;37:783-805.
6. Marschall J, Leone C, Jones M, et al. Catheter-associated bloodstream infections in general medical patients outside the intensive care unit: a surveillance study. Infect Control Hosp Epidemiol. 2007;28:905-9.
7. NHSN. National Healthcare Safety Network (NHSN) Surveillance Definitions. [online] Available from http://www.msic-online.org/pdf/NHSN_Definitions_CLABSI.pdf [Accessed December 2018].
8. Trick WE, Vernon MO, Welbel SF, et al. Unnecessary use of central venous catheters: the need to look outside the intensive care unit. Infect Control Hosp Epidemiol. 2004;25:266-8.

CHAPTER 26

Catheter-associated Urinary Tract Infections

Narayanappa D

Q1. What is an urinary catheter?

It is a drainage tube that is inserted into the urinary bladder through the urethra, is left in place, and is connected to a closed collection system. Other method that can be used is intermittent (in-and-out) catheterization involving brief insertion of a catheter into the bladder through the urethra to drain urine, this is used at intervals. Alternative methods when catheterization is not feasible or desirable are: an external catheter is a urine containment device that fits over or adheres to the genitalia and is attached to a urinary drainage bag, e.g. condom catheter or a suprapubic catheter which is surgically inserted into the bladder through an incision above the pubis.

Q2. What is the incidence of catheter-associated urinary tract infection (CAUTI)?

Catheter-acquired urinary infection is the source for about 20% of episodes of healthcare-acquired bacteremia in acute care facilities, and over 50% in long-term care facilities.

Q3. What is an urinary tract infection (UTI)?

An UTI is an infection that involves any of the organs or structures of the urinary tract, including the kidneys, ureters, bladder, and urethra. It presents as burning or pain in the lower abdomen, fever, burning micturition or an increase in the frequency of micturition.

Q4. What is the pathophysiology of CAUTI?

Either by intraluminal ascension or extraluminal ascension, organism reaches the urinary tract, preferred mechanism during CAUTI is extraluminal, where the organism ascends along the interface of catheter and urethra.

Q5. What are the risk factors for CAUTI?

Females, prolonged catheterization, impaired immunity, and lack of antimicrobial exposure are the common risk factors. Catheter blockage and low albumin levels are also considered.

Q6. Can CAUTIs be treated?

Yes, most CAUTIs are treatable with antibiotics and/or removal or change of the catheter.

Q7. What is the difference between CA-ASB and CAUTI?

CA-ASB is catheter-associated asymptomatic bacteriuria, usually by 30 days nearly all patients develop CA-ASB, but not CAUTI. About 25% of patients with CA-ASB might eventually develop CAUTI. CA-ASB does not need to be treated due to the risk of emergence of resistance, so it is crucial to differentiate both, which is decided by presence or absence of clinical features.

Q8. Define CAUTI.

Infectious Diseases Society of America (IDSA) definition: Urine growing more than or equal to 10^3 CFU/mL of more than or equal to one species in a patient with indwelling catheter or whose catheter has been removed in the last 48 hours who also has signs or symptoms of UTI.

Q9. What are the symptoms and signs of UTI?

Neonates present with jaundice, fever, failure to thrive, poor feeding, irritability, and vomiting.

Infants (2 months to 2 years) present with new onset or worsening of fever, rigors, altered mental state, malaise or lethargy with no other identified cause, irritability, vomiting, flank pain, costovertebral angle tenderness, and foul smelling urine.

Children above 2 years present with fever, vomiting, pain abdomen, increased frequency, urgency of micturition, and burning while micturition, acute hematuria, pelvic discomfort, and those whose catheters have been removed present with dysuria, urgency, frequency, and suprapubic pain or tenderness.

Q10. What is Centers for Disease Control and Prevention (CDC) definition of CAUTI?

Clinical features of UTI in a patient who has been catheterized for at least past 48 hours or whose catheter has been removed in the last 48 hours and whose urine sample either has:

- Growth greater than or equal to 10^5 CFU/mL of less than or equal to 2 species
- Growth greater than or equal to 10^3 to smaller than 10^5 CFU/mL of less than or equal to 2 species and has a positive urine analysis, i.e. positive dipstick for leucocytes/nitrite, pyuria or microorganisms on Gram stain.

Q11. What is National Healthcare Safety Network (NHSN) definition of CAUTI?

One or more of the following, with no alternate source:

- Fever
- Rigors (shaking chills)
- New onset hypotension with no alternate noninfectious cause
- New onset confusion/functional decline and increased leukocytosis
- New costovertebral angle pain or tenderness
- New or increased suprapubic pain or tenderness
- Acute pain, tenderness, or swelling of the testes, epididymis, or prostate
- Pus around the catheter insertion site.

And any of the following:

- If catheter removed within past 2 calendar days:
  - Clean catch (voided) urine culture with no more than 2 species of microorganisms, at least 1 of which is bacteria of 100,000 or more colonies (≥105 CFU/mL)
  - In/out catheter urine culture with any number of microorganisms, at least 1 of which is bacteria of 100 or more colonies (≥102 CFU/mL)
- If indwelling urinary catheter in place:
  - Positive urine culture with any number of microorganisms, at least 1 of which is bacteria of 100,000 colonies or more (≥105 CFU/mL).

Q12. What are features of UTI?

At least one of the following:

- Unexplained fever (>38°C)
- Costovertebral/ suprapubic pain/tenderness
- In those whose catheter is removed – dysuria, frequency, and urgency

For below or of 1 year of age, at least one of following:

- Fever (>38°C)
- Hypothermia (<36°C)
- Apnea
- Bradycardia
- Dysuria
- Lethargy or vomiting.

Q13. What is CA-ASB?

The IDSA and CDC define it as:

- Urine sample growing more than or equal to 10^5 CFU/mL of less than or equal to 2 species in an asymptomatic patient with indwelling catheter
- It is removed as separate infection now by CDC.

Q14. What is ideal method of collection of urine sample?

- *In a catheterized child*: Fresh sample should be collected before starting or changing antibiotics.
- *If plan is to replace a catheter*: Sample should be taken from new catheter, not the old one.
- *If no catheter*: Midstream voided sample is taken.
- Bagged sample, condom catheter sample not in use.

Q15. Catheter when to remove and when not to remove?

- Evidence states catheter can be changed in a suspected CAUTI, if catheter is more than 2 weeks old.
- Send culture from new catheter if replaced.
- If culture is positive, catheter should be ideally replaced if not done earlier.

Q16. What are the most common organisms of CAUTI?

Escherichia coli is the most common organism, others are *Klebsiella, Pseudomonas,* coagulase-negative staphylococci (CoNS), and *Enterococcus. Candida* is the most common fungus. Single pathogen is common.

Long-term catheters are associated with polymicrobial infections. *Proteus mirabilis* is an organism of unique importance in those with chronic indwelling catheters.

Q17. What is the choice of antibiotic?

- It is based on the pattern and sensitivity of local flora.
- *E. coli* is the most common organism, others are *Klebsiella, Pseudomonas,* CONS, and *Enterococcus. Candida* is the most common fungus. Single pathogen is common.
- BL/BLI like Piperacillin—Tazobactam (100 mg/kg/dose TID)
- If extended spectrum beta-lactamase (ESBL)—carbapenem like Meropenem (40–60 mg/kg TID)
- If enterococci—ampicillin and gentamycin
- If CONS—cloxacillin or vancomycin based on sensitivity patterns
- Monotherapy is sufficient usually.
- Duration of treatment depends on severity and response to treatment.
- 7 days in those with good response and 10–14 days in others. Uncomplicated UTI with catheter being removed, short course of 3 days may be considered.

Q18. How to prevent CAUTI?

- Reduce inappropriate use of catheters
- Consider alternatives for indwelling catheters wherever appropriate like condom catheters

- Antibiotic-coated catheters may be considered in immunocompromised
- Routine change of catheter, irrigation, prophylactic systemic antibiotics, meatal topical antibiotic, placing antiseptic solutions in the bag, and surveillance urine culture are not indicated.
- Daily in rounds the requirement of catheter should be questioned and should be removed promptly if no necessity is there.

Q19. What are the appropriate indications for indwelling catheter use?

- In case of acute urinary retention or bladder outlet obstruction.
- In critically ill patients, especially when comatose, for strict monitoring of urine output/hematuria.
- Perioperative use for selected surgical procedures:
- Patients undergoing urologic surgery or other surgery on contiguous structures of the genitourinary tract.
- Anticipated prolonged duration of surgery or patients anticipated to receive large volume infusions or diuretics during surgery or need for intraoperative monitoring of urinary output [these should be removed once shifted to intensive care unit (ICU)].
- To assist in healing of open sacral or perineal wounds in incontinent patients.
- Patient requires prolonged immobilization (e.g. potentially unstable thoracic or lumbar spine, multiple traumatic injuries such as pelvic fractures).
- To improve comfort in end of life care if needed.

Q20. What are inappropriate uses of indwelling catheters?

- As a substitute for nursing care of the patient
- For obtaining urine for culture or other diagnostic tests when the patient can voluntarily void
- As a part of prolonged postoperative care without appropriate indications (e.g. structural repair of urethra or contiguous structures, prolonged effect of epidural anesthesia, etc.).

Q21. Who should receive catheters?

- Perioperative patients
- Incontinent patients
- Those with bladder outlet obstruction
- Those with spinal cord injury
- Those with myelomeningocele and neurogenic bladder.

CHAPTER 27

Methicillin-resistant *Staphylococcus aureus*

Dhanya Dharmapalan

Q1. What is methicillin-resistant *Staphylococcus aureus* (MRSA)?

Methicillin-resistant *Staphylococcus aureus* (MRSA) is a gram-positive coccus that is catalase positive and oxidase negative with a characteristic "bunch of grapes" appearance under the microscope due to the activity of the coagulase enzyme. MRSA is *S. aureus* that has acquired the methicillin-resistance gene, *mecA*, on a mobile genetic element called the staphylococcal cassette chromosome mec (SCCmec).

Q2. Which are the risk factors for MRSA infection?

Anyone can get MRSA on their body from contact with an infected wound or by sharing personal items, such as towels or razors, that have touched infected skin. MRSA infection risk is increased in places that involve crowding, skin-to-skin contact, and shared equipment or supplies. People including athletes, daycare and school students, military personnel in barracks, and those who recently received inpatient medical care are at higher risk. Prior use of antibiotic within last 3 months is an important risk factor.

Q3. What are the types of MRSA?

Two main types of MRSA have been identified. These are community-associated MRSA (CA-MRSA) and healthcare-associated MRSA (HA-MRSA). Differences between them are as under **(Table 1)**.

Table 1: Differences in CA-MRSA and HA-MRSA.

	HA-MRSA	*CA-MRSA*
Healthcare contact	Yes	No
Mean age at infection	Older	Younger
Skin and soft tissue infections	Uncommon	Common
Antibiotic resistance including clindamycin, cotrimoxazole and doxycycline	Usually susceptible to clindamycin, cotrimoxazole or doxycycline	Some agents
Resistance gene	SCCmec types I, II, and III	SCCmec Type IV and V
Strain type	USA100 and 200	USA 300 and 400
PVL (Panton-Valentine leukocidin) toxin gene	Rare	Frequent

Q4. What is the clinical spectrum with MRSA infections?

It has a very wide spectrum, ranging from asymptomatic carrier to serious and often fatal systemic infections. It includes:

- Asymptomatic carrier
- Skin and soft tissue infections:
  - Impetigo
  - Cellulitis
  - Abscesses
  - Deeper soft tissue abscesses
  - Cervical lymphadenitis
  - Otitis externa and otitis media
  - Acute mastoiditis
- Severe and invasive infections:
  - Necrotizing pneumonia and empyema
  - Septic shock
  - Toxic shock syndrome
  - Musculoskeletal infections including pyomyositis
  - Osteomyelitis
  - Necrotizing fasciitis—more common in adults
  - Purpura fulminans
  - Disseminated infections with septic emboli and deep vein thrombosis.

Q5. What are the various antibiotics available to treat MRSA infections?

Community-acquired MRSA though resistant to all beta-lactam antimicrobial agents are usually susceptible to drugs like trimethoprim-sulfamethoxazole, clindamycin, and doxycycline.

The hospital-acquired MRSA usually harbor more resistant determinants and are only susceptible to vancomycin, linezolid, tigecycline or daptomycin.

As an empirical choice in sick children suspected with MRSA bacteremia, vancomycin should be used as first-line agent. Treatment should be tailored as per culture sensitivity reports. Clindamycin should be tested for inducible clindamycin resistance using the D-test.

Daptomycin is not approved for use in children less than 1 year due to its potential adverse effects on neuromuscular system. Tigecycline is a bacteriostatic agent, being a tetracycline compound should be avoided in children less than 8 years.

Ceftaroline has been recently approved for treatment of complicated MRSA skin and soft tissue infections in children above 2 months.

Q6. What is the management of MRSA skin and soft tissue infection?

Mild epidermal infections like impetigo and ecthyma can be treated by topical applications like mupirocin/retapamulin twice a day for 5 days. If numerous lesions, oral antibiotics clindamycin/doxycycline or cotrimoxazole can be used.

Mild MRSA purulent infections like abscess/furuncle require drainage alone. Moderate purulent skin infections like abscess/furuncle with systemic signs can be empirically treated after drainage with cotrimoxazole or doxycycline. Severe infections, i.e. those with systemic inflammatory response like fever of more than 38°, tachycardia, tachypnea, leucopenia or leukocytosis, or are immunocompromised should be empirically treated with vancomycin/linezolid in addition to drainage.

Nonpurulent infections like cellulitis can be treated with clindamycin in case of mild-to-moderate infections and vancomycin should be given in severe cases. For polymicrobial infections like necrotizing fasciitis, vancomycin is the first-line agent in addition in addition to gram-negative coverage. Surgical debridement of the infection is crucial step in management.

Ceftaroline and telavancin are new drugs on the block for treatment of complicated MRSA skin and soft tissue infections. Ceftaroline has been recently approved for treatment of complicated MRSA skin and soft tissue infections in children above 2 months.

Q7. What is the treatment for MRSA osteomyelitis/septic arthritis?

Surgical debridement with drainage of associated soft tissue abscess is essential in case of MRSA osteomyelitis or drainage of joint space is required for MRSA septic arthritis. If CA-MRSA is sensitive to clindamycin, it is the first-line treatment due to its very good penetration in the bones with switch oral from parenteral to oral clindamycin. But for clindamycin resistant bone and joint infections, parenteral therapy with vancomycin/daptomycin/linezolid with oral switch to linezolid is recommended. The duration of treatment is for at least 8–12 weeks.

Q8. How is MRSA meningitis managed?

Methicillin-resistant *Staphylococcus aureus* meningitis should be treated with vancomycin for at least 14 days in pediatric patients and 21 days in neonates.

Surgical drainage should be promptly done of any local abscess and there should be prompt removal of any infected ventriculoperitoneal (VP) shunt. The shunt should not be replaced unless repeated cerebrospinal fluid (CSF) cultures are sterile. Some experts recommend adding rifampicin (20 mg/kg/day in two divided doses).

Other alternative agents are cotrimoxazole (12 mg/kg/day of trimethoprim component). Linezolid being bacteriostatic should be avoided.

Q9. What is the treatment of MRSA pneumonia?

Methicillin-resistant *Staphylococcus aureus* pneumonia can be treated with vancomycin/linezolid/clindamycin (if sensitive). Meta-analysis of randomized controlled trials comparing linezolid or vancomycin in treatment of suspected MRSA pneumonia did not show evidence of superiority of either.

Use of antitoxin agent with linezolid/clindamycin may be necessary in necrotizing pneumonia. Empyema if present should be drained. Linezolid can also be used as oral switch therapy from vancomycin.

Tigecycline is not approved for use in less than 8 years of age and is not recommended for nosocomial/hospital-acquired MRSA infections. Daptomycin should not be used to treat pneumonia due to MRSA.

Q10. How is MRSA bacteremia/right-sided infective endocarditis (IE) treated?

Vancomycin or daptomycin, both being bactericidal are to be used in bacteremia or in MRSA endocarditis. Vancomycin is first-line treatment for neonatal MRSA bacteremia.

Linezolid/clindamycin being bacteriostatic are not recommended in these situations.

Q11. What is the treatment for MRSA-associated toxic shock syndrome?

Antitoxin agents like clindamycin/linezolid should be added to vancomycin in management of MRSA toxic shock syndrome.

Q12. How can vancomycin therapy be optimized?

Vancomycin should be dosed at 15 mg/kg 6 hourly. The target trough levels 15–20 μg/mL in children. Serum trough concentrations should be obtained at steady state conditions, prior to the fourth or fifth dose of vancomycin. The monitoring of trough levels is recommended for critically ill children and those with serious infections.

Q13. What are the side effects of vancomycin?

Vancomycin infusion can cause anaphylaxis. Red man syndrome can occur due to rapid infusion of the first dose of the drug. It causes urticaria and erythematous rash over head, neck, and upper torso due to histamine release. In this situation vancomycin should be stopped and diphenhydramine administered. Vancomycin is nephrotoxic. Renal function should be monitored during its use.

Q14. What are the side effects of linezolid?

Linezolid can commonly cause diarrhea and abnormal liver function tests. Treatment with longer duration (more than 2 weeks) is associated with bone marrow toxicity, lactic acidosis, optic neuropathy, and peripheral neuropathy. Weekly monitoring of complete blood count (CBC) is required while on linezolid.

Q15. What are the characteristics of daptomycin?

Daptomycin is a bactericidal agent. It is an alternative to vancomycin in bacteremia, right-sided IE, osteomyelitis, and skin and soft tissue infections. It has adverse effects of raised creatine phosphokinase (CPK) levels, myopathy, and peripheral neuropathy. It is not Food and Drug Administration (FDA) approved in less than 1 year of age.

Q16. What is advised for recurrent MRSA infections?

Methicillin-resistant *Staphylococcus aureus* abscess, if present, should be drained and treated with antibiotics. Possible sources like foreign bodies/ devices/implants must be removed. Child should be investigated for underlying immunodeficiency.

Decolonization with MRSA decolonization with mupirocin applied twice a day for 5 days plus a skin antiseptic solution (e.g. chlorhexidine for 5–14 days or dilute bleach baths). There are concerns about safety of antiseptics in neonatal age group and till more data emerges, these should be preferably avoided. Personal items such as towels, sheets, and clothes should be decontaminated.

Q17. How MRSA infection spread can be prevented?

- Maintain good hand and body hygiene.
- Wash hands often and clean your body regularly, especially after exercise.
- Keep cuts, scrapes, and wounds clean and covered until healed.
- Avoid sharing personal items such as towels and razors.
- Prompt medical attention for suspected infective lesion.

FURTHER READING

1. Liu C, Bayer A, Cosgrove SE, et al. Clinical practice guidelines by the Infectious Diseases Society of America for the treatment of methicillin-resistant Staphylococcus aureus infections in adults and children. Clin Infect Dis. 2011; 52(3):e18-55.
2. Stevens DL, Bisno AL, Chambers HF, et al. Practice guidelines for the diagnosis and management of skin and soft tissue infections: 2014 update by the Infectious Diseases Society of America. Clin Infect Dis. 2014;59(2):e10-52.
3. UpToDate. (2018). Bacterial meningitis in children older than one month: Treatment and prognosis. [online] Available from https://www.uptodate.com/contents/bacterial-meningitis-in-children-older-than-one-month-treatment-and-prognosis [Accessed December 2018].
4. UpToDate. (2018). Hematogenous osteomyelitis in children: Management. [online] Available from https://www.uptodate.com/contents/hematogenous-osteomyelitis-in-children-management [Accessed December 2018].
5. US FDA. (2018). New Pediatric Labeling Information Database. [online] Available from https://www.accessdata.fda.gov/scripts/sda/sdNavigation.cfm?sd=labelingdatabase&displayAll=true [Accessed December 2018].
6. Wang Y, Zou Y, Xie J, et al. Linezolid versus vancomycin for the treatment of suspected methicillin-resistant *Staphylococcus aureus* nosocomial pneumonia: a systematic review employing meta-analysis. Eur J Clin Pharmacol. 2015;71(1):107-15.

CHAPTER 28

Extended-spectrum Beta-lactamases

Vijay Yewale

Q1. What are beta-lactamases?

Beta-lactamases are enzymes produced by bacteria inactivating penicillin and narrow spectrum cephalosporins such as cephalexin and cefazolin. Higher generation cephalosporins like cefotaxime, ceftriaxone, ceftazidime, and cefepime are not inactivated by beta-lactamases. These oxyimino-cephalosporins were widely used in treatment of beta-lactamase producing organisms.

Q2. What are extended-spectrum beta-lactamases (ESBLs)?

The effectiveness of oxyimino-cephalosporins was short lived as bacteria produced ESBLs that could inactivate higher generation cephalosporins. They cannot inactivate cefoxitin, cefotetan, and carbapenems. ESBL can also be overcome by beta-lactamases like sulbactam, clavulanate, and tazobactam combined with a beta-lactam line piperacillin and cefoperazone.

Q3. Which organisms produce ESBLs?

Extended-spectrum beta-lactamases have been found exclusively in gram-negative organisms, primarily in *Klebsiella pneumoniae, Klebsiella oxytoca,* and *Escherichia coli* but also in *Acinetobacter, Burkholderia, Citrobacter, Enterobacter, Morganella, Proteus, Pseudomonas, Salmonella, Serratia,* and *Shigella* species.

Q4. What are the types of beta-lactamases?

TEM, SHV, CTX-M, and OXA are the different types of beta-lactamases. Though not all, most are ESBLs. OXA beta-lactamases are mainly found in *Pseudomonas aeruginosa.* OXA beta-lactamases with carbapenemase activity have also been described. There are a few other less common types of ESBLs found in *Pseudomonas aeruginosa and Enterobacteriaceae.*

Q5. How are the ESBLs detected by the laboratories?

Extended-spectrum beta-lactamases are detected by their ability to confer resistance to oxyimino cephalosporins like cefotaxime, ceftriaxone, ceftazidime, and cefepime and the ability of clavulanic acid to inhibit them.

Q6. What is the prevalence of ESBLS?

Extended-spectrum beta-lactamase-producing *Enterobacteriaceae* have been reported worldwide, most often in hospital specimens, but also in samples from the community. Prevalence rates vary from hospital to hospital and from country to country.

Extended-spectrum beta-lactamases are found in many gram-negative bacteria causing infections both in the hospital settings and in the community today. The prevalence of ESBL in *E. coli* causing urinary tract infections (UTIs) from the community is in the range of 40–50%. Almost 70–80% of health care associated infections by gram-negative bacteria are with ESBL production.

There are sporadic reports of ceftriaxone resistance in *Salmonella* due to production of a new type of ESBL.

Q7. What are the risk factors for ESBL production?

- Colonization of the gastrointestinal (GI) tract with ESBL producing *Enterobacteriaceae*
- Prolonged hospital or intensive care unit (ICU) stay
- Hemodialysis
- Presence of intravascular catheter
- Prior use of antibiotic, especially third-generation cephalosporins.

Q8. What are the treatment options for ESBL infections?

Infections with ESBL-producing organisms are associated with higher mortality rates, longer hospital stays, greater hospital expenses, and reduced rates of clinical and microbiologic response compared with similar infections with gram-negative bacteria that do not produce ESBL.

Beta-lactam + beta-lactamase inhibitors

Piperacillin-tazobactam or cefoperazone-sulbactam show in vitro efficacy against ESBL producing organisms. Piperacillin-tazobactam is more effective against CTX-M type of beta-lactamase. There is limited data with the use of cefoperazone-sulbactam. However, high inoculum can lead to treatment failure. Secondly coproduction of other enzyme like AmpC beta-lactamase can also make treatment with beta-lactam/beta-lactamase agent unsuccessful. Several different types of beta-lactamases may be coproduced by the same bacteria making treatment challenging. Piperacillin-tazobactam is a good alternative in the treatment of UTI caused by ESBL organisms as it achieves higher concentrations in urine. Treatment with beta-lactam/beta-lactam inhibitor can be optimized by using higher doses, frequent dosing, and continuous infusion. Because of poor cerebrospinal fluid (CSF) penetration they are not recommended for ESBL intracranial infections.

Cefepime

Also exhibits inoculum effect. Mortality is higher with cefepime as compared to other agents. It is found to be more efficacious with minimum inhibitory concentration (MIC) less than 1 mg/L. Most isolates from India have MICs more than 1 mg/L. Cefepime + tazobactam is a promising agent, but there is not enough clinical trial data to recommend for treatment.

Carbapenems

Preferred agent (meropenem, imipenem, doripenem, and ertapenem) producing best outcomes and bacteriologic clearance. Meropenem and imipenem are equally effective and meropenem is preferred over imipenem for its best safety profile in children. Doripenem is relatively new agent and ertapenem has advantage of once daily dosing. Because of its excellent CSF penetration it remains an obvious choice of ESBL intracranial infection like neonatal meningitis.

Other agents

Tigecycline, a non-beta-lactam drug that is a potential alternative for treatment of ESBL-producing strains, especially for patients with beta-lactam allergies, although data on its clinical use for this purpose are limited.

Empiric therapy of ESBL infections

Empiric treatment is guided by:

- Degree of sickness of patient
- Local susceptibility patterns including in vitro resistance to beta-lactam/beta-lactam inhibitors especially in nosocomial infections
- Site of infection
- Host comorbidity
- Whether adequate source control is possible or not
- Carbapenem in severe infections
- Choice is difficult in less serious infections and therapy is guided by factors mentioned above
- The spread of ESBL-producing organisms within institutions can be slowed by the use of barrier protection and restriction of later generation cephalosporins.

CHAPTER 29

Carbapenem-resistant Enterobacteriaceae

Abhay K Shah

Q1. What are carbapenem-resistant enterobacteriaceae (CRE)?

Enterobacteriaceae are a family of gram-negative bacteria that are often found in our gastrointestinal tract (GIT) and are often responsible for infections both in community and healthcare settings. Enterobacteriaceae that are nonsusceptible to at least one of the carbapenem antibiotics and/or produce an enzyme (carbapenemase) that would make them resistant to carbapenem group of antibiotics are termed as CRE. In general they are resistant to almost all antibiotics.

The current modified definition from Centers for Disease Control and Prevention (CDC) for CRE surveillance includes resistant to imipenem, meropenem, doripenem, or ertapenem or documentation that the isolate possesses a carbapenemase. This will cover both carbapenemase-producing CRE (CP-CRE) and non-CP-CRE.

Q2. What are the mechanisms for carbapenem resistance?

- Intrinsic resistant bugs like *Stenotrophomonas maltophilia,* Proteus species, and Providencia species.
- Carbapenemase production:
  - *Klebsiella pneumoniae* carbapenemase (KPC): The genes that code for KPC are on a highly mobile genetic material and hence can be transmitted from one bacterium to another easily.
  - New Delhi metallo-beta-lactamase (NDM), Verona integron-encoded metallo-beta-lactamase (VIM), and imipenemase metallo-beta-lactamase (IMP). NDMs are more common in endemic healthcare settings.
- Porin mutation limiting carbapenems entry into the bacteria
- Porin loss
- Combination of more than one mechanism.

Q3. What is the importance of CRE?

- Enterobacteriaceae are a common cause of infections in both community and healthcare settings.

- They are resistant to multiple classes of antimicrobials and have limited therapeutic options.
- Genetic element encoding carbapenemases can be transmitted from one Enterobacteriaceae to another very easily and transmission of resistance is a constant threat.
- Associated with high mortality and prolonged hospital stays.

Q4. Which are the risk factors?
- Prior intensive care unit (ICU) admission
- Gastrointestinal tract or genitourinary surgery or procedure
- Prior antibiotic use.

Q5. Which are common infections encountered with CRE?
- Bloodstream infections
- Ventilator-associated pneumonia (VAP)
- Urinary infections
- Sepsis.

Q6. How do CRE get transmitted?
- Contact
- Surgical wounds
- Injury wounds
- Devices like catheters, intravenous (IV) lines, and ventilators.

Q7. What are therapeutic options for CRE?
- Colistin
- Tigecycline
- Fosfomycin
- Aminoglycosides
- Optimizing combination therapy (high-dose meropenem with adjuvant drug).

Q8. How will you optimize empiric treatment in suspected CRE?
This depends on site of infection, minimal inhibitory concentration (MIC) for carbapenems, previous antibiotic use, comorbid conditions, etc.

Site of infection	***Empiric core drug***	***Empiric adjuvant***	***Definitive***
Bloodstream	• High-dose meropenem or doripenem • Polymyxin B	• Aminoglycoside • Tigecycline • Fosfomycin • Rifampin	Use MIC Value
Lung	• High-dose meropenem doripenem • Polymyxin B	• Tigecycline • Aminoglycoside • Fosfomycin • Rifampin	

Contd...

Contd...

Site of infection	***Empiric core drug***	***Empiric adjuvant***	***Definitive***
GIT/biliary tract	• High-dose meropenem doripenem • Polymyxin B • High-dose tigecycline	• Fosfomycin • Rifampin	Use your MIC IQ
Urine	• High-dose meropenem doripenem • Fosfomycin or aminoglycoside	• Colistin • Aminoglycoside	

(GIT: gastrointestinal tract; IQ: inhibitory quotient; MIC: minimal inhibitory concentration)

Q9. How the antibiotic therapy can be guided after culture and sensitivity report?

- Do not use single agent
- Use combination therapy
- Do not ever forget to de-escalate
- Treatment should be guided by MIC values (see below) and not otherwise sensitivity report.

Meropenem/doripenem:

- MIC less than or equal to 16 µg/mL continue high-dose meropenem/ doripenem
- MIC more than 16 µg/mL consider alternative in vitro active antimicrobial

Polymyxin B/colistin:

- MIC less than or equal to 2 µg/mL continue polymyxin B/colistin
- MIC more than 2 µg/mL consider alternative in vitro active antimicrobial

If both meropenem/doripenem MIC (>16 µg/mL) and polymyxin B/ colistin MIC (>2 µg/mL), then consider a high-dose tigecycline-based regimen or a dual carbapenem-based regimen. If pandrug-resistant infection, select case-reports support dual carbapenem-based regimen.

Tigecycline:

- MIC less than or equal to 1 µg/mL consider tigecycline
- MIC more than 1 µg/mL consider alternative in vitro active antimicrobial

Fosfomycin:

- MIC less than or equal to 32 µg/mL consider fosfomycin
- MIC more than 32 µg/mL consider alternative in vitro active antimicrobial

Aminoglycoside:

- MIC less than or equal to 2 µg/mL (gentamicin/tobramycin) or less than or equal to 4 µg/mL (amikacin) consider aminoglycoside
- MIC more than 2 (gentamicin/tobramycin) or more than 4 µg/mL (amikacin) consider alternative in vitro active antimicrobial.

Q10. Which are newer agents for CRE?

Fosfomycin: It has activity against KPC-producing *K. pneumoniae* and New Delhi metallo-β-lactamase (NDM)-1-producing Enterobacteriaceae. Fosfomycin achieves high urinary concentrations for prolonged time periods and is mainly meant for MDR UTI as a component of combination therapy.

The combination cephalosporin-beta-lactamase inhibitor agents:

- Ceftolozane-tazobactam (C/T)
- Ceftazidime-avibactam

They are approved by Food and Drug Administration for complicated intra-abdominal infections (with metronidazole), complicated urinary tract infections. The addition of tazobactam to ceftolozane resulted in an improved activity compared to other antibiotics such as ceftazidime. In addition to excellent activity against *Pseudomonas aeruginosa*, it has very good in vitro activity against other important gram-negative organisms, such as *Escherichia coli* and *Klebsiella* pneumoniae. Given the current in vitro data C/T appears as a very promising anti-pseudomonas option.

SECTION 5

Salvaging the Antibiotics

CHAPTER 30

Antibiotic Stewardship

Shyam Kukreja

Q1. Why there is a need for antimicrobial stewardship (AMS) program?

Antimicrobial resistance is rapidly increasing; currently we are in an era of superbugs like methicillin-resistant *Staphylococcus aureus* (MRSA), carbapenem-resistant enterobacteriaceae (CRE), vancomycin-resistant *S. aureus* (VRSA), vancomycin-resistant enterococci (VRE), multiple-drug resistant (MDR), and extensively drug-resistant tuberculosis (XDR TB), etc. However, development of antimicrobial drugs has slowed down acutely. Now more than ever before, AMS is of utmost importance to optimize the use of antimicrobials and to slowdown the development of further resistance and improve patient outcomes.

Q2. What is the meaning of antimicrobial stewardship?

Steward means to manage or look after. "Antimicrobial stewardship" is being used more and more in recent years, generally referring to programs and interventions that aim to manage (optimize) antimicrobial use.

Q3. The term "stewardship" is not used in other clinical fields, for example, there is no "antihypertensive drug stewardship" or "diabetic drug stewardship". What is the reason?

The use of antimicrobials in individual ultimately affects the whole community. The misuse of antibiotic leads to development of resistance.

Antibiotics lose their efficacy over a period of time, e.g. most staphylococci which were once sensitive to penicillin are resistant today. While the efficacy of antihypertensive drug or diabetic drug is the same today as it was when the drug was developed.

Antimicrobials are the only class of drugs with potential clinical impact on both the treated individual as well as on community.

Antimicrobial stewardship is about using antimicrobials responsibly, which should balance both the individual's need for appropriate treatment and the long-term societal need for sustained access to effective therapy (Dyar et al., 2017). The definition of AMS has been evolving over the years.

Q4. What is the clinical impact of antimicrobials on the treated individual?
Unnecessary early-life antibiotic use in infants and children leads to alteration in their microbiota, which can become the cause of allergies, recurrent infections, autoimmune disorders, inflammatory bowel disease, and obesity.

Q5. What is the clinical impact of use of antimicrobial on community?
Misuse of antibiotics in individuals initiates development of resistance in bacteria by selection pressure. These resistant bugs then start circulating in the community. As a result, community starts getting infected by resistant bugs. So, misuse of antibiotics in individuals adversely impacts the health of individuals who are not even exposed to them (i.e. community). Therefore, there is a great need for responsible use of antibiotics.

Q6. What is the current definition of antimicrobial stewardship?
According to Centers for Disease Control and Prevention (CDC), antibiotic stewardship is the effort:
- To measure antibiotic prescribing
- To improve antibiotic prescribing by clinicians and use by patients so that antibiotics are only prescribed and used when needed
- To minimize misdiagnoses or delayed diagnoses leading to underuse of antibiotics
- To ensure that the right drug, dose, and duration are selected when an antibiotic is needed.

Q7. What are the goals of antibiotic stewardship?
The goal of antibiotic stewardship is to maximize the benefit of antibiotic treatment while minimizing harm to both individuals and communities.

Q8. What actions are to be done to achieve the objective of antibiotic stewardship?
Simply, clinicians should use antibiotics responsibly. Such clinicians are referred to as good antimicrobial stewards. In fact, patient should also act responsibly when prescribed antibiotics. Other antibiotic prescribers like farmers and veterinarians should also use antibiotics responsibly.

Q9. What all a clinician should do to become a good antimicrobial steward?
- Make accurate diagnoses
- Take cultures at appropriate times
- Follow local antimicrobial guidelines in management
- Ensure that right antibiotic is prescribed in the correct dose and for the correct duration
- Regularly review the need for therapy
- Inappropriate and unnecessary use of antimicrobials must be avoided.

Q10. How patient should act responsibly?

- Take antimicrobial courses as recommended by the doctor
- Not storing or using leftover antimicrobials
- No self-medication.

Q11. What are the barriers or road blocks in achieving the objective of antibiotic stewardship?

Inappropriate and unnecessary use of antimicrobials. In USA, it is estimated that approximately half of outpatient antibiotics prescribed in humans might be inappropriate, including unnecessary antibiotic prescription, incorrect antibiotic selection, dosing, or duration. At least 30% of outpatient antibiotic prescriptions in the United States are unnecessary. Improving antibiotic therapy is the prerequisite for AMS program.

In fact, the most important modifiable risk factor for antibiotic resistance is inappropriate prescribing of antibiotics.

Q12. Why would a clinician use inappropriate antibiotic?

- These might include clinician's knowledge gaps about clinical practice guidelines
- Perceived pressure to see patients quickly
- Clinician's concerns about decreased patient satisfaction when antibiotics are not prescribed
- Patient demanding antibiotic prescription.

A prerequisite before implementing antibiotic stewardship interventions is that clinicians must use all opportunities to improve antibiotic prescribing.

Q13. What are the benefits of antibiotic stewardship?

- Improved patient outcomes
- Reduction in development of antibiotic resistance
- Decrease in cost of treatment
- Decrease in adverse drug resistance
- Decrease in antibiotic-associated disease, e.g. antibiotic-resistant diarrhea, oral candidiasis, and *Clostridium difficile* associated diarrheas
- Nonalteration of the patient's microbiome including the gut flora, respiratory tract flora, urogenital tract flora, and skin flora
- Prevention of environmental degradation.

Q14. How can AMS program be developed in hospitals?

There are six core elements of antibiotic stewardship in a hospital. These are:

1. A single leader [preferably infectious disease (ID) specialist] responsible for outcomes
2. A single pharmacy leader

3. Tracking of antibiotic use
4. Regular reporting of antibiotic use and resistance
5. Educating providers on use and resistance
6. Specific improvement interventions.

   Antimicrobial stewardship programs are almost nonexistent in India.

Q15. What about implementing AMS in outpatients?

In developed countries, approximately 80–90% of antibiotic use occurs among outpatients. In India, there is much higher consumption of antibiotics in outpatient department (OPD) practice and misuse of antibiotics. There is a greater need to have AMS programs in outdoor practice in India.

Q16. How can AMS program be implemented in office practice?

According to CDC:

- *Commitment of prescriber*: Demonstrate dedication to and accountability for optimizing antibiotic prescribing and patient safety.
- *Action for policy and practice*: Implement at least one policy or practice to improve antibiotic prescribing, e.g. commit not to prescribe antibiotic for acute watery diarrheas and watery nose.
- *Tracking and reporting*: Monitor antibiotic prescribing practices, e.g. in self-evaluate antibiotic prescribing practices (more so in India because of no systematic electronic record keeping).
- *Education and expertise*: Provide educational resources to clinicians and patients on antibiotic prescribing.

Continuing medical educations (CMEs), guidelines by Indian Academy of Pediatrics (IAP), Infectious Diseases Society of America (IDSA), etc. would be helpful for clinicians to improve their antibiotic prescription. The book in your hand is also an attempt to achieve the same objective.

CHAPTER 31

Infection Control in Healthcare Settings

Bhaskar Shenoy

Q1. What are the healthcare-associated infections (HCAIs) and how are they transmitted?

Healthcare-associated infections are those acquired at any point in time during the care provided in the healthcare system. These infections may be transmitted in many ways (respiratory tract, digestive tract or by contact), but the way they are most often transmitted is by hand contact by healthcare workers.

Q2. How significant is the problem of infections in healthcare across the world?

Healthcare-associated infections occur worldwide and affect hundreds of millions of patients both in developed and developing countries. Lack of reliable and standardized surveillance data suggests a significant underestimation of the real burden of disease.

The risk of acquiring HCAI is universal and pervades every healthcare facility and system around the world. Healthcare workers are often the conduit for the spread of such infections to other patients in their care. It should also be noted here that many patients may carry microbes without any obvious signs or symptoms of an infection (colonized or subclinically infected). This clearly reinforces the need for hand hygiene, irrespective of the type of patient being cared for.

Q3. What is hand hygiene?

Hand hygiene is understood as being a procedure for the purpose of reducing the number of microorganisms on the skin of one's hands. When this procedure is performed with soap and water, it is termed handwashing. When it is performed with an alcohol-based preparation or with antiseptic soap, it is called hand disinfection.

Q4. Which is better, washing or disinfecting your hands?

When one's hands are soiled, they should be washed with soap and water, given that soap facilitates eliminating soiling. When one's hands are contaminated, but are not visibly soiled, the procedure of choice is disinfection using alcohol-based preparations, given that antiseptics eliminate a greater number of microorganisms.

Q5. Why is hand hygiene important?

Because it is the simplest and most effective way we all have of preventing the spread of infections transmitted by contact. Different publications show hand hygiene to contribute to reducing HCAIs.

Q6. When must hand cleansing be performed?

Always before and after coming into contact with anyone requiring care at any point in the health system. The World Health Organization (WHO) additionally recommends the following:

- Always before performing a clean/aseptic procedure.
- Always after there have been any possibility of contact with body fluids.
- Always after contact with the patient's surroundings.

Q7. Who must perform hand cleansing?

All healthcare workers involved in caring for patients, independently of whatever the patients diagnoses may be. Hand hygiene must also be performed by the patients, their family members, and the visitors caring for them.

Q8. How is hand hygiene performed?

Figure 1 describes how hand hygiene is performed.

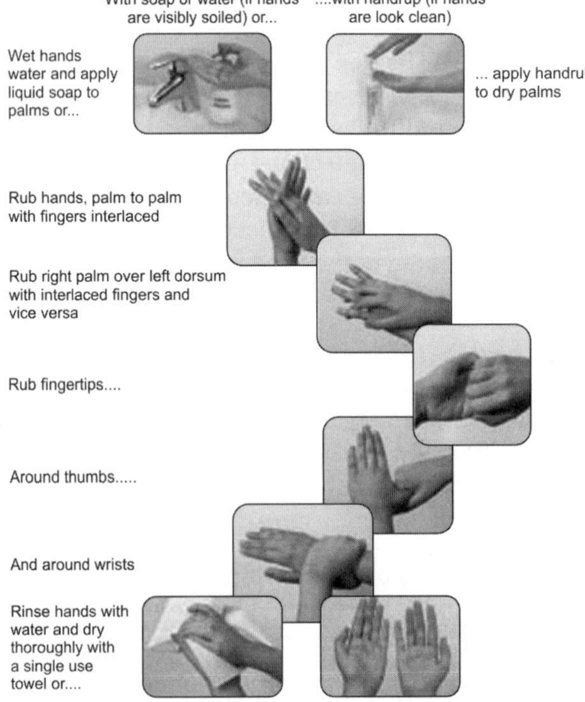

Fig. 1: Steps of hand hygiene.

Q9. How long does it take to perform hand cleansing?

For handwashing, one's hand should be rubbed with soap and water for 15 seconds, plus the length of time necessary for rinsing, and then drying. Hand rubbing with alcohol-based preparations must be continued until hands are thoroughly dry. The amount of preparation used must allow one to rub one's hands for at least 15 seconds. If the manufacturer were to recommend a longer time, the manufacturer's instructions must always be followed.

Q10. What factors must be taken into account to prevent damaging the skin on one's hands?

To prevent skin problems, it is very important that one's hands been perfectly dry on completing the procedure. After washing with soap and water, the necessary paper towels must be used to ensure that one's hands are thoroughly dry. Similarly, when cleansing with an alcohol-based preparation, one must rub one's hands until the preparation has completely dried. It is advisable for healthcare workers to take care of their hands by moisturizing them several times a day, preferably after finishing work for the day.

Q11. Can wearing gloves be a substitute for hand cleansing?

No, never. Gloves can in no case be a substitute for hand cleansing. If gloves are worn, they must always be changed between one patient and the next, and every time they are removed.

Q12. What types of microbes can spread due to lapses in hand hygiene?

The following are examples of the types of microbes that can be spread on the hands of healthcare workers:

- *Staphylococcus aureus* [including methicillin-resistant *S. aureus* (MRSA)]
- *Streptococcus pyogenes* (group A streptococcus)
- Vancomycin-resistant enterococci (VRE)
- *Klebsiella* [including extended spectrum beta-lactamases (ESBL)-producing *Klebsiella*]
- *Escherichia coli* (including ESBL-producing *E. coli*)
- *Enterobacter* species
- *Pseudomonas* species [including multidrug-resistant (MDR) *Pseudomonas* species)
- *Clostridium difficile*
- *Candida* species.
- *Rotavirus*
- *Adenovirus*
- Hepatitis A virus
- *Norovirus.*

Wounds contain large numbers of microbes. Areas around the perineum can be heavily loaded with microbes, but even the armpit, trunk, and hands can be frequently covered in huge numbers. Microbes such as *S. aureus* and *Klebsiella* can be present on intact skin in numbers ranging from 100 to 1,000,000 per square cm.

Q13. How important are clean hands in the overall patient safety agenda?
Hand hygiene contributes significantly to keeping patients safe. It is a simple, low-cost action to prevent the spread of all microbes that cause HCAI. While hand hygiene is not the only measure to counter HCAI, compliance with it alone can dramatically enhance patient safety, because there is much scientific evidence showing that microbes causing HCAI are most frequently spread between patients on the hands of health-care workers.

Q14. What are the commodities required to implement the WHO guidelines on hand hygiene in healthcare?

Consumables:

- Alcohol-based handrubs (either locally produced or a commercial product compliant with WHO recommendations)
- 100 mL alcohol-compatible plastic bottles for the handrub (pocket carriage by health-care workers)
- Non-medicated liquid soap. Alternatively, non-medicated bar soap (small bars) with soap racks to facilitate drainage
- Dispensers for liquid soap
- Antimicrobial soap for surgical hand scrub
- Single-use hand towels
- Creams or lotions for skin care (they should not interfere with the antimicrobial action of handrub)
- Medical gloves—single use examination gloves for routine patient care
- Medical gloves—sterile surgical gloves.

Other items:

- Sinks
- Clean running water
- 500 mL wall-mounted dispensers for alcohol-based handrub
- Printed material.

Q15. What does "point of care alcohol-based handrub" mean in practice?
Making alcohol-based handrub available at the point of care means making it available at the exact place where care or treatment involving physical contact between a patient and a health-care worker takes place. Point-of-care products should be accessible without leaving the patient environment.

This enables health-care workers to make hand hygiene habitual and quickly and easily take action to ensure compliance in relation to the indications corresponding to the "My 5 Moments for Hand Hygiene" approach, thus killing the pathogens and preventing their spread.

It is important to understand that the product must be capable of being used without leaving the patient zone. Point-of-care is usually achieved through health-care worker-carried handrubs (pocket bottles) or handrubs fixed to the patient's bed, bedside table or to the wall next to the patient's bed. Handrubs affixed to an object, e.g. trolleys, or dressing or medicine trays which are taken into the patient environment, can also fulfill this definition, if they are reliably taken into the patient zone in anticipation of contact.

Q16. What is respiratory hygiene/cough etiquette?

These are infection prevention measures designed to limit the transmission of respiratory pathogens spread by droplet or airborne routes. The strategies target primarily patients who may have undiagnosed respiratory infections.

Q17. What are the elements of respiratory hygiene?

- Implement measures to prevent the spread of respiratory infections from anyone in a healthcare setting with signs or symptoms.
    - Post signs at entrances asking patients with symptoms of respiratory infection to:
        - Cover your mouth and nose when coughing or sneezing.
        - Use tissues and throw them away.
        - Wash your hands or use a hand sanitizer every time you touch your mouth or nose.
    - Provide tissues and no-touch receptacles for their disposal.
    - Provide resources for performing hand hygiene in or near waiting areas.
    - Offer masks to symptomatic patients when they enter the healthcare setting.
    - Provide space and encourage symptomatic patients to sit as far away from others as possible. Facilities may wish to place these patients in a separate area, if available, while waiting for care.
- Educate healthcare personnel (HCP) on the importance of prevention measures when examining and caring for patients with signs and symptoms of a respiratory infection.

Q18. Describe respiratory hygiene/cough etiquette.

The following measures to contain respiratory secretions are recommended for all individuals with signs and symptoms of a respiratory infection.

- Cover your mouth and nose with a tissue when coughing or sneezing;

- Use in the nearest waste receptacle to dispose of the tissue after use;
- Perform hand hygiene (e.g. handwashing with nonantimicrobial soap and water, alcohol-based handrub, or antiseptic handwash) after having contact with respiratory secretions and contaminated objects/materials.

Healthcare facilities should ensure the availability of materials for adhering to respiratory hygiene/cough etiquette in waiting areas for patients and visitors.

- Provide tissues and no-touch receptacles for used tissue disposal.
- Provide conveniently located dispensers of alcohol-based handrub; where sinks are available, ensure that supplies for handwashing (i.e. soap and disposable towels) are consistently available.

Masking and separation of persons with respiratory symptoms: During periods of increased respiratory infection activity in the community (e.g. when there is increased absenteeism in schools and work settings and increased medical office visits by persons complaining of respiratory illness), offer masks to persons who are coughing. Either procedure masks (i.e. with ear loops) or surgical masks (i.e. with ties) may be used to contain respiratory secretions (respirators such as N-95 or above are not necessary for this purpose). When space and chair availability permit, encourage coughing persons to sit at least three feet away from others in common waiting areas. Some facilities may find it logistically easier to institute this recommendation year-round.

Q19. What do you mean by the term "universal precautions (UPs)"?

The term UP refers to the standards of infection control developed to prevent exposure and transmission of blood-borne infectious agents like human immunodeficiency virus (HIV) and hepatitis virus. The UP should be implemented and practiced at all times by all healthcare providers and caregivers in all settings, in particular in hospitals, health centers, health posts and community settings, as well as in the homes of patients.

Q20. Why are UPs needed?

Universal precautions were developed because it is not possible to identify all patients with blood-borne diseases caused by microorganisms. Increased risks are faced by healthcare workers when providing care to HIV-positive patients, or those infected with other blood-borne agents such as the hepatitis virus. The term "universal" reflects the fact that they are intended to refer to contact with *all* patients, not just those known to have blood-borne infections.

Universal precautions are designed to provide for the safe handling of infectious material, including amniotic fluid, cerebrospinal fluid, pleural fluid, abdominal fluid, serum, semen, vaginal fluids, and blood and blood-tainted body fluids. As part of this process, barriers to infection were developed, such as gloves, gowns, masks, and eye goggles to protect health workers from splashes or sprinkles of infectious materials. Safety involves not just patient contact, but the management of the environment in which the patient is situated. With UPs, everyone is considered infectious, since it is impossible to tell ahead of time who is infected and who is not.

Q21. What is safe injection practice?

A common source of injury for healthcare workers is poor practice when giving injections. These are standard procedures for giving an injection, designed to ensure safety of healthcare workers and that of patients when giving injections in the health post and in the patient's home.

Q22. Preparing to give an injection.

Using a new sterile syringe and needle for each injection is one of the most effective ways to prevent the spread of blood-borne infections.

- Use a new packaged sterile syringe and needle for *every* injection.
- Inspect the packaging very carefully. Discard a needle or syringe if the package has been punctured, torn or damaged in any way.
- Check the expiry date on the package. Never use needles or associated injection materials that are "out of date".
- Prepare injections in a clean designated area or on a clean surface; in a patient's home you will need to use a clean dish or tray that you have washed in soap and water, left to air dry and then swabbed with alcohol before laying out the injection equipment.
- Prepare each dose immediately before administering; do not prepare several syringes in advance.
- Do not touch the needle. Discard a needle that has touched a nonsterile surface.

Q23. What is needle-stick injury?

A *needle-stick injury* refers to a healthcare worker accidentally puncturing their own skin with a needle that has previously been used to inject a patient. Needle-stick injuries can occur at any time, but they happen most frequently during and immediately after an injection are given. They can also occur when needles are not disposed of in safety boxes, for example when a healthcare worker picks up contaminated waste in which a needle has been left unnoticed.

In general, the more injection equipment that is handled, the greater the risk of needle-stick injuries. *But these injuries are preventable.*

Q24. What are the steps to reduce the risk of needle-stick injuries?

- Handle needles and syringes as little as possible; avoid recapping the needle after use, and do not remove a used needle from the syringe.
- Handle needles and syringes safely; ensure you wear suitable gloves, and avoid recapping needles.
- Setup the injection preparation area so as to reduce the risk of injury.
- Position the patient, especially children, correctly for injections.
- Place a safety box close to where the injections are being given, so that used syringes and needles can be disposed of immediately. Practice safe disposal of all contaminated sharps and waste.

Q25. What care should be taken while recapping used needles?

Although you should not recap needles routinely, you may need to recap a needle to avoid carrying an unprotected sharp when immediate disposal is not possible, or if an injection is delayed because a child is agitated. If it does become necessary for you to recap a used needle, follow the *one-handed recapping* technique (also called the *single-handed scoop* method) **(Fig. 2)**.

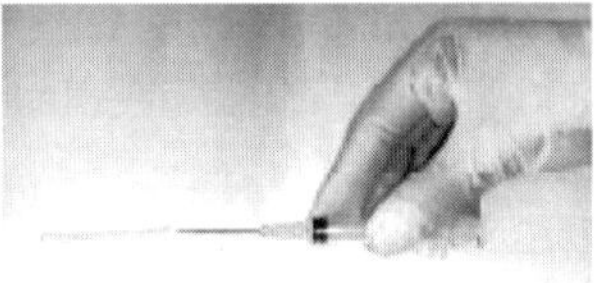

Step 1
Place the cap on a flat surface, then remove your hand from the cap

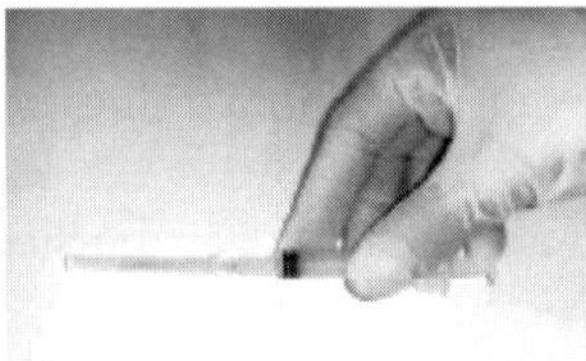

Step 2
With one hand, hold the syringe and use the needle to 'scoop up' the cap.

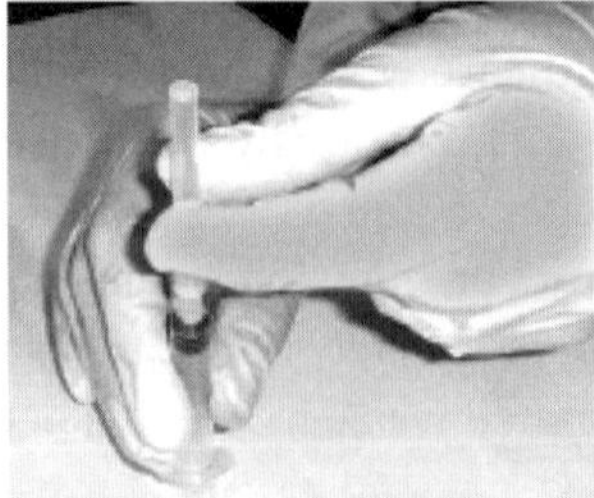

Step 3
When the cap covers the needle completely, use the other hand to secure the cap on the needle hub. Be careful to handle the cap at the bottom only.

Fig. 2: The "one-handed" technique for recapping a needle.

Q26. What does occupational exposure mean?

Occupational exposure means coming in contact with infectious agents whilst carrying out duties as a healthcare worker.

Examples of occupational exposure to HIV are needle-stick or other sharps injuries, a splash of infected body fluid into the eyes or onto cracked skin, bites, and sexual assaults by infected patients. Procedures such as gynecological examinations, spinal taps, labor and delivery, and surgery can also place the health worker at risk. Splash exposure carries a lower risk than a needle-stick injury, but it should be taken seriously in both the workplace and the patient's home. The risk of transmission of HIV after accidental occupational exposure is about *100 times less* than the risk of occupational transmission of the hepatitis B virus.

Q27. Why should the HIV test be repeated at intervals up to 6 months after the exposure?

It takes up to 3 months before the body of a person newly infected with HIV produces enough anti-HIV antibodies to be detectable in an HIV rapid test. This is called the *"window period"*. A negative test result during this period cannot be taken as evidence that the exposure did not transmit HIV.

Q28. What is droplet precaution?

Droplet precautions include wearing a surgical or procedure mask for close contact, in addition to standard precautions, when examining a patient with symptoms of a respiratory infection, particularly if fever is present. These precautions should be maintained until it is determined that the cause of symptoms is not an infectious agent that requires *droplet precautions.*

Q29. What are the measures to contain MRSA infection?

Hand hygiene: Healthcare personnel can transmit organism acquired by touching the contaminated surfaces of environment or patient. This is one of the best defense against MRSA infection. Alcohol handrub should be available at every bed of patient.

Gloves and mask: Must be worn for invasive procedure contact with sterile sites all activities which are at risk of exposure to blood or body fluids.

Gloves and mask should be removed after contact and disposed safely according to standard biowaste protocol.

Environment sanitation:

- Cleaning and disinfectant protocol to be followed strictly.
- All reusable equipment should be cleaned and disinfected.

Antibiotics stewardship: Injudicious use of vancomycin and linezolid should be avoided to prevent emergence of resistance.

Management of patient infected with methicillin-resistant S. aureus:

- Physical isolation has the advantage of interrupting transmission to other

- Clean and disinfect reusable medical equipment
- Linen and clinical of the patient needs to be transported in a sealed bag and incinerated movement of patient in hospital to be minimized.

Staff screening: Screening of HCP indicated if transmission of MRSA continuous despite active control measure.

Decolonization:

- It helps to prevent infection in MRSA carriers as well as transmission to noncarrier population.
- Decolonization therapy includes application of mupirocin to anterior nares two to three times a day for 5 days.

Skin decolonization: Using 4% chlorhexidine body wash, 7.5% povidone-iodine is useful.

Education of all HCP and family members of patient.

Q30. What are the infection control precautions to be followed in office practice?

Recommendation for infection control in waiting area:

- Waiting room should be adequately ventilated
- Ideally six air exchange/hour
- Facility for handwash/alcoholic handrub
- Patient with communicable disease should triaged and immunocompromised patient to be given priority
- Regular cleaning of floors and surfaces in the waiting area through wet mopping
- Visible soiling by vomitus, urine, and feces should be promptly cleaned, followed by disinfectant
- Toys should be washed with soap and water daily
- Educational poster for respiratory adequate and hand hygiene to be displayed.

Recommendation for infection control inside clinician chamber:

- Hand hygiene
- Use alcohol-based handrub after examination of each patient.

Maintenance of reusable medical equipments:

- Stethoscope, otoscope, and infantometer are low risk of infection transport
- Washing with soap and water is adequate
- Clinical thermometer should be washed with soap water or wiped with 70–90% ethyl or isopropyl alcohol
- Disposable tongue depressor or recommended.

Equipment for personal safety:

- Gloves and mask should be used, before any invasive procedure or where there is risk of exposure to body fluids
- After use needle should not be recapped
- Needle should be disposed in puncture proof closed container.

Immunization: All HCP should be vaccinated against hepatitis B and recommended to be immunized against measles, mumps, varicella, influenza, and tetanus.

Education and training of staff: Biowaste management should be done as per the infection management and environment plan policy by Indian ministry of health.

Q31. How to prevent transmission of tuberculosis (TB) in household?

- Proper and adequate ventilation in house
- Cough etiquette and respiratory hygiene to be followed
- Smear positive TB patient to be isolated in properly ventilated room
- Should spend minimal time in public transport and large gatherings
- Chemoprophylaxis for children below 6 years with isoniazid (INH)
- Prevention from culture positive MDR-TB in household
- Practice cough etiquette and respiratory hygiene
- Healthcare personnel should wear respirators while attending infectious MDR-TB cases.

Q32. What precaution to be taken to prevent risk of transmission from H1N1 patient?

- Standard precautions: Contact airborne droplet to be followed
- Standard precaution should apply to immunocompromised patient
- *Environmental control*: Cleaning and disinfection
- Droplet precaution include use of personal protective equipment (PPE), patient placement, and patient transport in personal protection medical mask should be used if working within 1 meter of the patient
- Patient should be placed in single room or in cohort
- Patient movement should be limited and patient should wear medical mask when outside their room
- *Contact precautions*:
  - PPE and hand hygiene
  - Patient placement and transport
- Chemoprophylaxis
- Immunization.

SECTION 6

Annexures

Annexure I: Antibiotic Dosages

Jeeson C Unni

Table 1: Antibiotic Dosages

Name	*Formulations*	*Dosage and interval*
Penicillins A. Penicillinase susceptible Amoxicillin	Inj: 250, 500 mg. Cap/Tab/DT: 125, 250, 500 mg. Syr: 125, 250 mg/5 mL Drp: 100 mg/mL	Oral 20–50 mg/kg/day in 2 or 3 divided doses. Higher dose of 80–90 mg/kg in acute suppurative otitis media (maximum of 500 mg 2–3 times daily). In uncomplicated gonorrhea: 3 g with 1 g probenecid.
Ampicillin	Inj: Vial 250, 500, 1,000 mg. Cap/Tab/DT: 125, 250, 500 mg. Syr: 125, 250 mg/5 mL. Drp: 100 mg/mL	Neonate: 50 mg/kg/dose <7 days 12th hrly, 7–21 days 8th hrly, >21 days 6th hrly. 100 mg/kg/dose for suspected meningitis and group B streptococcal infection. Children: Oral 1 month to 2 yrs 12.5 mg/kg/dose, 2–12 yrs 250 mg/dose and 12–18 yrs 500 mg/dose; IV/IM 25 mg/kg/dose (maximum 1 g/dose); IV infusion 100 mg/kg/dose (maximum 3 g/dose) - all given 4 times daily.
Penicillin G	Inj: 500,000 units/vial (300 mg) Tab: 200,000, 400,000, 800,000 units 600 mg = 1,000,000 units (1 MU) or 1 unit = 1,666 mg	Given IV. In newborn 25 mg (approx 40,000 units)/kg/dose 2 times daily up to 7 days of age and 3 times daily thereafter. Dose is doubled in meningitis. In children 25 mg/kg/dose 4 times daily. Double dose is given in meningitis 6 times daily to a maximum single dose of 2.4 g (approx 40 L units) and a maximum daily dose of 14.4 g (approx 2.3 crores units).
Phenoxymethylpenicillin	Tab: 125 mg 250 mg	Oral 250 mg/day, 1–5 yr 500 mg/day, 6–12 yr 1 g/day and 12–18 yr 2 g/day (severe infection 3 g/day) in 4 divided doses. Pneumococcal infection prophylaxis: Half the above daily dose in 2 divided doses. Rheumatic fever prophylaxis: 500 mg/day in 2 divided doses.

Contd...

Contd...

Name	***Formulations***	***Dosage and interval***
Benzathine penicillin	Inj: 600,000 units, 12,000,000 units and 24,000,000 units	Infants and children: Group A streptococcal URI—25,000–50,000 units/kg as single dose, max 12 L units/dose or child < 27 kg, 3–6 L units as single dose and > 27 kg, 9 L units as single dose. Adolescents 12 L units as single dose Prophylaxis of rheumatic fever: IAP recommends: Children < 27 kg 6 lakh units every 15 days; ≥27 kg 1.2 lakh units every 21 days. Congenital syphilis: 50,000 units/kg/dose (max 24 L units) once a week for 3 weeks. Early syphilis in adolescents: 24 L units as single dose in 2 injection sites. If present for > 1yr: 24 L units as single dose in 2 injection sites once weekly for 3 doses.
B. Penicillinase-resistant Cloxacillin	Inj: 250, 500 mg. Cap: 250, 500 mg. Syr: 125 mg/5 mL	Newborn IV/oral <7 days 50–100 mg/kg/day in 2 divided doses; 7–21 days 75–150 mg/kg/day in 3 divided doses, > 21 days 100–200 mg/kg/day in 4 divided doses. May be increased to 100 mg/kg/dose in severe infection (meningitis, cerebral abscess, staphylococcal osteitis). Oral used only for minor infections. Children: IV/IM 50–100 mg/kg/day in 4 divided doses (max single dose 1 g, may be doubled in severe infection) Oral < 1 yr 250 mg/day, 1–5 yr 500 mg/day, 5–18 yr 1 g in 4 divided doses. Doses may be doubled in severe infection. In renal failure if creatinine clearance < 10 mL/minute/1.73 m^2, increase dosage interval to 8th hrly.

Contd...

Contd...

Name	**Formulations**	**Dosage and interval**
C. Penicillins with beta-lactamase inhibitors Amoxicillin-clavulanate	Inj: (amoxicillin + clavulanate) 1,000 + 200, 500 + 100, 250 + 50 Tab: 500 + 125, 400 + 57, 250 + 125, 200 + 28.5 Syr: 400 + 57, 200+28.5, 125+31.25	Dosed on amoxycillin content. Neonates 30 mg/kg/day in 2 divided doses. Children 20–45 mg/kg in 2–3 divided doses. Higher doses of 80 mg/kg/day may be required in otitis media. Administration: Oral: give at the start of a meal. Dispersible tablets should be stirred into a little water before taking. IV: reconstitute a 600 mg vial with 10 mL Water for injections (final volume 10.5 mL) and a 1.2 g vial with 20 mL (final volume 20.9 mL). Give by slow IV injection (over 3–4 minutes, within 20 minutes of reconstitution) or infuse over 30–40 minutes and complete infusion within 4 hrs of reconstitution. For infusion the reconstituted injection can be diluted to 5 times its volume in NaCl 0.9%. Do not infuse in glucose solutions, as co-amoxiclav is less stable in infusions containing glucose.
Ampicillin–sulbactam	Inj: Ampicillin 1,000, 500 + Sulbactam 500, 250. Tab: Ampicillin 220 + sulbactam 147	Calculated on ampicillin IV N: 50 mg/kg bd. 1–4 weeks 37.5–50 mg/kg qds. > 4 weeks 50–100 mg/kg qds. Oral: 15 mg/kg qds. M = 12,000 mg
Piperacillin-tazobactam	Vials 2,000 mg piperacillin + 250 mg tazobactam; 4,000 mg piperacillin + 500 mg tazobactam	Dosed on piperacillin component Newborn IV 90 mg/kg/dose 3 times daily Children IV 90 mg/kg/dose 4 times daily (max single dose 4.5 g).
Cephalosporins First-generation Cephalexin	Cap/Tab/DT: 125, 250, 500 mg. Syr: 125, 250 mg/5 mL Drp: 100 mg/mL	Children 25–100 mg/kg/24 hrs in 3–4 divided doses; adolescent 250–500 mg 4 times daily (maximum 4 g/24 hr. Reduce dose in severe renal impairment (creatinine clearance < 10 mL/minute/1.73 m^2) by reducing dose frequency. Removed by dialysis thus an additional dose may be required after dialysis.

Contd...

Contd...

Name	***Formulations***	***Dosage and interval***
Cefadroxil	Cap/Tab/DT: 125, 250, 500 1,000 mg. Syr: 125, 250 mg/5 mL Drp: 100 mg/mL	Children orally 30 mg/kg/24 hrs in 2 divided doses (maximum 2 g/day); adolescent 250–500 mg 8th–12th hrly.
Cefazolin	Vials: 125, 250, 500, 1,000 mg	12.5–25 mg/kg qds M = 12,000 mg
Cephalosporins Second-generation Cefaclor	Tab/DT/Cap: 250, 375, 500 mg Syr: 125, 187.5, 250 mg/5 mL Drp: 50 mg/mL	Orally < 1 yr 62.5 mg, 1–5 yr 125 mg, 6–18 yr 250 mg/dose 3 times daily. Dose doubled in severe infection with susceptible organisms.
Cefuroxime ,	Inj: Vials 500, 750, 1,500 mg Tab: 125, 250, 500, 750 mg Syr: 125 mg/5 mL	Infections due to sensitive gram-positive and gram-negative bacteria: Orally (as cefuroxime axetil) 3 months to 2 yr 10 mg/kg (max 125 mg) twice daily; 2–12 yrs 15 mg/kg (max 250 mg) twice daily; 12–18 yrs 250 mg twice daily; double the dose for severe lower respiratory tract infections; 125 mg twice daily in lower urinary tract infection (UTI). IV, IV infusion, IM <7 days age: 25 mg/kg 12 hrly; 7–21 days age 25 mg/kg 8 hrly; 21–28 days age: 25 mg/kg 6th hrly; severe infection in neonates give IV at double these doses. 1 month to 18 yrs 20 mg/kg (max 750 mg) 8 hrly; increase to 50–60 mg/kg (max 1.5 g) 6–8 hrly in severe infection and cystic fibrosis. Lyme disease: Orally 3 months to 12 yr 15 mg/kg (max 500 mg) bd for 14–21 days (for 28 days in Lyme arthritis); 12–18 yrs 500 mg bd for 14–21 days (for 28 days in Lyme arthritis). Surgical prophylaxis: IV 1 month to 18 yrs 50 mg/kg (max 1.5 g) up to 30 minutes before procedure; up to 3 more doses of 30 mg/kg (max 750 mg) may be given IM/IV 8 hrly for high-risk procedures.

Contd...

Contd...

Name	***Formulations***	***Dosage and interval***
Cephalosporins Third-generation Cefotaxime	Inj: Vial 125, 250, 500, 1,000, 1,500 mg	Newborn (severe infections like meningitis) 50 mg/kg/dose: <7 day 2 times, 7–21 day 3 times, 21–30 days 3–4 times. 1 month to 12 yr 50 mg/kg/dose and 12–18 yr 1–3 g 2 times daily. Dosage adjustment in renal impairment due to extrarenal elimination. It is only necessary to reduce dose in severe renal impairment (creatinine clearance < 10 mL/minute/1.73 m^2). A normal single dose should be given as a loading dose then the daily dose should be halved without a change in frequency.
Ceftriaxone	Inj: Vial 100, 125, 200, 250, 500, 750, 1,000, 2,000 mg	Neonates 50–75 mg/kg once daily IM/IV. Infuse over 10–30 minutes. Avoid in premature, acidotic or hyperbilirubinemic neonates. Children 50–75 mg/kg once daily IV/IM. Meningitis loading dose 75 mg/kg followed by 80–100 mg/kg/24 hrs once or divided 12 hrly. Maximum 4 g/day. In severe renal failure reduce dose to a maximum of 2 g or 50 mg/kg. No dose adjustment required in hepatic impairment. If both hepatic and severe renal impairment monitor serum concentrations. In patients undergoing dialysis no supplemental dose required but serum concentration monitoring advisable.
Ceftizoxime	Vials 200, 1,000 mg	Child 30–50 mg/kg tds M = 12,000 mg

Contd...

Contd...

Name	Formulations	Dosage and interval
Ceftazidime	Vials 250, 500, 1,000 mg	Neonates < 7 days and > 7 days < 1,200 g 100 mg/kg/24 hrs in 2 divided doses IV/IM, > 7 days > 1,200 g 150 mg/kg/day divided 8th hrly IM/IV. Children 150 mg/kg/24 hrs divided 8th hrly. Maximum 6 g/day. Single dose > 1 g to be given IV only. Dose adjustment in renal failure: In mild impairment give a dose very 12 hrs, in moderate impairment (creatinine clearance 10–50 mL/minute/1.73 m^2) give a dose once daily and in severe impairment (creatinine clearance < 10 mL/minute/1.73 m^2) give 50% of dose once daily. Levels may be monitored if clinically indicated. In hemodialysis: the appropriate maintenance dose should be repeated after dialysis. In peritoneal dialysis: 125–250 mg may be added to 21 of dialysis fluid, and given in addition to the IV dose.
Cefoperazone	Vials: 250, 500, 1,000, 2,000 mg	50–200 mg/kg/day in 2 or more divided doses (max in adolescent 1–2 g IM/IV 12th hrly)
Cefixime	Tab/DT: 100, 200, 400 mg. Syr: 50 mg/5 mL, 100 mg/5 mL	8 mg/kg/24 hrs in 1–2 divided doses; adolescent: 400 mg/24 hrs in 1–2 divided doses. Typhoid: Oral cefixime is used in a dose of 15–20 mg per kg per day in two divided doses.
Cefpodoxime	Tab/DT: 50, 100, 200 mg Syr: 50, 100 mg/5 mL	9 mg/kg/day in 2 divided doses (maximum single dose: 200 mg). The dose frequency should be reduced in renal impairment. Creatinine clearance 10–40 mL and < 10 mL/minute/1.73 m^2, frequency of dosing once in 24 hrs and once in 48 hrs respectively.
Cefdinir	Cap/Tab: 300 mg Syr: 125 mg/5 mL	14 mg/kg/day in 2 divided doses.

Contd...

Contd...

Name	***Formulations***	***Dosage and interval***
Cephalosporins Fourth-generation Cefepime	Inj: 250, 500, 1,000, 2,000 mg	Neonates <14 days 30 mg/kg/dose twice daily IV/IM. Neonates >14 days 50 mg/kg/dose twice daily IV/IM. Children IV 50 mg/kg every 8 hrs (maximum 2 g/dose). Intraperitoneal 15 mg/kg/dose. In peritoneal dialysis associated with peritonitis 1,000 mg/24 hrs. However, not yet licensed for use in children under 12 yr in UK and US.
Monobactams Aztreonam	Vial: 250, 500, 1,000, 2,000 mg	IV over 3–5 minutes or IV infusion < 7 day old 30 mg/kg 12th hrly; rest of neonatal period and up to 12 yr 30 mg/kg 6–8th hrly. In severe infection and cystic fibrosis in 2–12 yr olds may increase up to 50 mg/kg 6–8th hrly (max 2 g 6th hrly); 12–18 yr 1 g 8th hrly or 2 g 12th hrly (severe infection with *P. aeruginosa* or pulmonary infection in cystic fibrosis). Renal impairment: CrCl 10–30 mL/minute/1.73 m^2, no change in first dose but subsequent doses to be halved; CrCl < 10 mL/minute/1.73 m^2, no change in first dose but subsequent doses to be reduced to 1/4th usual dose.
Glycopeptides, lipopeptides Vancomycin	Vials: 500, 1,000 mg	Drug of choice in MRSA, *Clostridium jeikeium* and for serious infections in penicillin allergic patients. Newborn: IV 15 mg/kg/dose < 28 weeks once daily, 29–35 weeks twice daily and > 35 weeks 3 times daily. Intrathecal all newborn 2.5–5 mg once daily. Child IV 15 mg/kg loading dose followed by 10 mg/kg/dose 4 times daily (max 2 g/day). Intrathecal 1 month to 4 yr 5 mg, 4–15 yr 10 mg and > 15 yr 20 mg once daily. Children with enlarged ventricles need higher doses. Adjust dose according to CSF levels aiming for a trough level of < 10 mg/L. Pseudomembranous colitis: Oral vancomycin at 40 mg/kg/day divided q 6–8 hrs for 7–10 days; not to exceed 2 g/day.

Contd...

Contd...

Name	***Formulations***	***Dosage and interval***
Teicoplanin (Teichomycin A)	Vials: 200, 400 mg	*Newborn*: Loading 16 mg/kg and 24 hrs later start maintenance 8 mg/kg/day as single dose; children 10 mg/kg/dose 2 times daily × 3 doses and then once daily in same dose for severe infection and 6 mg/kg/day once for mod infection. Orally for pseudomembranous colitis 10 mg/kg/dose 2 times daily. May be given intraventricular and intraperitoneal.
Daptomycin	Vials: 350 mg	Adequate data in children not available Should be used only as salvage drug For skin and soft tissue 4 mg/kg IV OD For endocarditis and bacteremia 6–8 mg/kg (up to 12 mg/kg)
Sulfonamides Cotrimoxazole	Tab: *(trimethoprim content)* 20 mg, 40 mg, 80 mg, 160 mg. Syr: 40 mg/5 mL *(with Sulfamethoxazole in ratio of 1:5)*	*Dosed on trimethoprim*: *Children*: Orally 6–20 mg TMP/kg/24 hrs divided 12th hrly (maximum 160 mg TMP 12th hrly). *P. carinii* pneumonia oral/IV 15–20 mg TMP/kg/24 hrs divided 12th hrly. *P. carinii* prophylaxis orally 5 mg TMP/kg/24 hrs or 3 times/week. The use of co-trimoxazole is not generally recommended under 6 weeks of age, but some neonatologists feel that there is no specific reason for this caution other than the risk of hemolytic anemia in babies with G6PD deficiency and the risk of kernicterus because sulfamethoxazole competes for the protein binding sites usually available to bilirubin in babies with jaundice. If co-trimoxazole is used in newborn infants it is given in the same dosage as for 6 weeks to 5 months but trimethoprim on its own is now usually preferred to co-trimoxazole.

Contd...

Contd...

Name	***Formulations***	***Dosage and interval***
Silver sulfadiazine	Skin cream 1%, Eye drops 1%	*Burns*: After cleaning the wound apply over all affected areas to a depth of 3–5 mm, using a sterile gloved hand or sterile spatula. Where necessary, reapply to any area from which it has been removed by patient activity. Reapply at least every 24 hrs or more frequently if the volume of exudates is large. *Hand burns*: Apply to the burn and enclose the whole hand in a clear plastic bag or glove which is then closed at the wrist. The patient should be encouraged to move the hand and fingers and the dressing should be changed when an excessive amount of exudates has accumulated in the bag. *Leg ulcers/pressure sores*: The cavity of the ulcer should be filled with cream to a depth of at least 3–5 mm, followed by application of an absorbent pad or dressing, with further application of pressure bandaging as appropriate. Dressings should be changed daily, but if less exudates every 48 hrs may be sufficient. *Fingertip injuries*: Hemostasis of the injury should be achieved prior to the application of a 3–5 mm layer of cream, and then the finger covered with a finger dressing or the finger of a plastic glove. Dressings should be changed every 2–3 days. In all cases, use the contents of the tube or pot on one person only. Discard 50 g tubes 7 days after opening. Discard 250 g and 500 g pots 24 hrs after opening.

Contd...

Contd...

Name	*Formulations*	*Dosage and interval*
Quinolones Nalidixic acid	Tab/DT: 125, 250, 500, 1,000 mg. Syr: 300 mg/5 mL	Urinary tract infection due to susceptible organisms: Oral: Adolescents: 1 g suspension or tablet PO every 6 hrs for 1–2 weeks. Maintenance dose of 500 mg PO every 6 hrs. Children and infants ≥ 3 months: The recommended total daily dosage for initial therapy is 55 mg/kg/day PO, administered in four equally divided doses. For prolonged therapy, the total daily dose may be reduced to 33 mg/kg/day PO. UTI prophylaxis in children: Oral: Children and infants ≥ 2 months to 2 yrs: A dose of 30 mg/kg/day PO in two divided doses has been recommended. Maximum dosage limits: Adolescents: 4 g/day PO. Children and infants ≥ 3 months: 55 mg/kg/day PO. Infants < 3 months: Safe and effective use has not been established. Patients with hepatic impairment: Exercise caution when using nalidixic acid in patients with liver disease, however, no specific dosage adjustments are indicated. Patients with renal impairment: Decrease the dose by half in patients with a CrCl less than or equal to 20 mL/minute.
Norfloxacin	Tab/DT: 100, 200, 400, 800 mg. Syr: 100 mg/5 mL. Drp: 10 mg/mL Eye drops 0.3%	6–10 mg/kg bd M = 800 mg

Contd...

Contd...

Name	***Formulations***	***Dosage and interval***
Ciprofloxacin	Tab: 200, 250, 400, 500, 750 mg. Inj: 2 mg/mL 100 mL bottle Eye drops 0.3%	Neonates 10 mg/kg 12 hrly orally or IV; children 15–30 mg/kg/24 hrs in 2 divided doses oral or IV (maximum single dose IV 400 mg and oral 750 mg). Dose adjustment in renal or liver failure: In severe impairment (creatinine clearance < 20 mL/minute/1.73 m^2) total daily dosage may be reduced by half, although monitoring serum levels provides the most reliable basis for dose adjustment. No adjustment in impaired hepatic function. Corneal ulcers: Apply throughout the day and night. First day: 2 drops every 15 minutes for 6 hrs followed by 2 drops every 30 minutes for the rest of the day. 2nd day: 2 drops every hour and from 3rd to 14th day: 2 drops 4th hrly. Superficial infections of eye: 1–2 drops 4 times daily till 48 hrs after the eye is clinically normal (use for max of 21 days).
Ofloxacin	Tab/DT: 50, 100, 200, 400 mg. Syr 50 mg/5 mL Inj: 2 mg/mL 100 mL bottle. Eye drops 0.3%	Eye drops: > 1 yr 1 drop 2–4 hrly for 1st 48 hrs and then 4 times daily till 2 days after healing is achieved (max 10 days). Ear drops: Otitis externa 1–12 yr 5 drops and 12–18 yr 10 drops to affected ear(s) 2 times daily for 10 days. CSOM: > 12 yr 10 drops to affected ear(s) 2 times daily for 14 days. AOM with perforation or with tympanostomy tubes 1–12 yr: 5 drops to affected ear(s) 2 times daily for 10 days. IV and oral: 10–15 mg/kg/day in a single dose or divided twice daily. Systemic use: It is replaced by levofloxacin which is an S-isomer of ofloxacin and has less side effects.

Contd...

Contd...

Name	*Formulations*	*Dosage and interval*
Levofloxacin	Tab: 250, 500, 750 mg. Inj: 5 mg/mL 100 mL bottles	Pediatric dose not established 10 mg/kg has been used M = 750 mg
Nadifloxacin	Skin cream 0.1%	Apply bd
Aminoglycosides Streptomycin	Vials: 750, 1,000 mg	Tuberculosis: IM daily regimen 15 mg/kg as single morning dose (range 15–20 mg/kg; max dose 1 g/day); intermittent regimen 15 mg/kg (range 15–20 mg/kg).
Gentamicin	Inj: Vials 40 mg/mL and 10 mg/mL Amp: 20, 40, 60, 80 mg Eye drops 0.3%	Many dose regimens exist for aminoglycosides depending on target concentration aimed for and patient groups treated. The dose regimens shown here are generally accepted initial doses and dose adjustments should be made in the light of serum concentration measurement. Neonates IV/IM < 7 days 1,200–2,000 g 2.5 mg/kg once in 12–18 hrs and >2,000 g 2.5 mg/kg once in 12 hrs; > 7 days 1,200–2,000 g 2.5 mg/kg once in 8–12 hrs and >2,000 g 2.5 mg/kg once in 8 hrs. Extended interval dose regimen by slow intravenous injection or intravenous infusion: < 32 weeks gestation 4–5 mg/kg every 35 hrs; > 32weeks gestation 4–5 mg/kg every 24 hrs. Children: <12 yr 7.5 mg/kg/day and 12–18 yr 3–6 mg/kg/day in 3 divided doses. Plasma levels done after 3–4 doses to achieve predose level of < 2 mg/L and 1 hr postdose peak of 5 mg/L. Alternatively 5–7.5 mg/kg/24 hrs IV once daily. Plasma levels done 18–24 hrs after 1st dose to achieve predose level of < 1 mg/L and 1 hr postdose peak of 16–20 mg/L. Once daily dose regimen (not for endocarditis or meningitis) by intravenous infusion: Child 1 month to 18 yrs: initially 7 mg/kg, then adjusted according to serum-gentamicin concentration. Intrathecal/ventricular preservative free preparation: Newborn 1 mg/24 hrs; children 1–2 mg/24 hrs; 16–18 yr. Pseudomonal lung infection in cystic fibrosis: By inhalation of nebulized solution; child 1 month to 2 yrs 40 mg twice daily; child 2–8 yrs 80 mg twice daily; child 8–18 yrs 160 mg twice daily. 0.3% eye drops: 1–2 drops up to 6 times/day. In severe infections 1 drop every 15–20 minutes and gradually decreasing frequency as infection gets controlled till 48 hrs after healing. 1.5% eye drops for severe eye infection. Ear drops: 2–3 drops 3–4 times daily and at night; children and adults.

Contd...

Contd...

Name	***Formulations***	***Dosage and interval***
Netilmicin	Amp: 50 mg/mL; 100 mg/mL 2, 3 mL ampoules	Newborn IV 3 mg/dose 12th hrly. Increase to 8th hrly after 1 week age postnatal. Monitor after 3rd dose for 1 hr postdose peak of 8–12 mg/L and a trough of <3 mg/L. Prolong dose interval in PDA, prolonged hypoxia and indomethacin therapy. Children: IV/IM <12 yr 7.5 mg/kg/day and > 12 yr 6 mg/kg/day in 3 divided doses or 1 month; 18 yr 7.5 mg/kg as single dose daily. Intraperitoneal 7.5–10 mg/L in peritoneal dialysis fluid.
Amikacin	Inj: 50 mg/mL, 125 mg/mL, 250 mg/mL	Many dose regimens exist depending on target concentration aimed for and patient groups treated. The doses mentioned are accepted initial doses and dose adjustments done depending on serum levels. Newborn: loading dose of 10 mg/kg then 7.5 mg/kg every 12 hrs IV < 35 weeks up to 14 days 10 mg/kg once daily and >14 days 10 mg/kg loading dose followed by 7.5 mg/kg/dose 2 times daily; >35 weeks < 14 days 15 mg/kg as single dose daily and > 14 days 10 mg/kg loading dose followed by 7.5 mg/kg/dose 2 times daily. Extended interval dose regimen by slow intravenous injection or intravenous infusion: 15 mg/kg every 24 hrs. Children (1 month to 18 yrs): IV/IM 7.5 mg/kg/dose 2 times daily up to maximum of 500 mg/dose. Child > 12 yrs with life-threatening infection: 1.5 g/day in 3 divided doses for up to 10 days may be given. Aim for 1 hr postdose (peak) of 15–30 mg/L. Once daily dose regimen (not for endocarditis or meningitis): Child 1 month to18 yrs, initially 15 mg/kg, then adjusted according to serum-amikacin concentration.
Neomycin	Cap: 350 mg. Oint: 2%	Adolescents: 0.25–1 g four times. Children: 12.5 mg/kg/dose oral in diarrhea and 3 g/m^2/day q 6 hrs. oral in hepatic coma. Eye drops: Superficial eye infection 1 drop 2–4 times daily, severe infection 1 drop every 15–20 minutes initially then reducing frequency as infection gets controlled. Eye ointment: 3–4 times daily. Treatment to continue till 2 days after condition is cured.

Contd...

Contd...

Name	***Formulations***	***Dosage and interval***
Tobramycin	Vials: 2 mL each; 10, 30, 40 mg/mL Eye Oint: 0.3% Drp: 0.3%	Newborn: IV < 32 weeks 4–5 mg/kg 36 hrly and > 32 weeks 4–5 mg/kg once in 24 hrs. PDA, prolonged hypoxia, indomethacin treatment necessitate increased dose intervals. Extended interval dose regimen by intravenous injection over 3–5 minutes or by intravenous infusion: Neonate less than 32 weeks postmenstrual age 4–5 mg/kg every 36 hrs; neonate 32 weeks and over postmenstrual age 4–5 mg/kg every 24 hrs. Child: IV/IM 2.5 mg/kg/dose 3 times daily or 7 mg/kg as single daily dose. Once daily dose regimen by intravenous infusion. Child: 1 month to18 yrs, initially 7 mg/kg, then adjusted according to serum-tobramycin concentration. Pseudomonal lung infection in cystic fibrosis: Child 1 month to 18 yrs, 8–10 mg/kg/daily in 3 divided doses. Once daily dose regimen by intravenous infusion over 30 minutes. Child 1 month to 18 yrs, initially 10 mg/kg (max 660 mg), then adjusted according to serum-tobramycin concentration. Chronic pulmonary *Pseudomonas aeruginosa* infection in patients with cystic fibrosis. By inhalation of nebulized solution: Child 6–18 yrs, 300 mg every 12 hrs for 28 days, subsequent courses repeated after 28 days interval without tobramycin nebulizer solution. Intraventricular: newborn 1 mg/day, child 1–2 mg/day, adolescent 2–4 mg/day. Eye drops 1 drop 2 hrly and then reduce frequency as infection is controlled. To continue till 2 days after healing.
Framycetin	Eye drops: 1% Oint: 5%	Eye drops: 1–2 drops 2 hrly and reducing gradually as infection gets controlled to 48 hrs after the eye is clinically normal. Eye ointment: 3 times daily when given alone or at bedtime along with eye drops given during the day. Cream: Apply 1–3 times daily.

Contd...

Contd...

Name	***Formulations***	***Dosage and interval***
Macrolides Erythromycin	Cap/Tab/DT: 125, 250, 333, 500 mg. Syr: 100, 125, 250 mg/5 mL Drp: 100 mg/mL Eye Oint 0.1% Oint, lotion, gel, 2%, 3%, 4%	General indications: Neonates: Orally/IV < 7 days age 20 mg/kg/day 2 times daily; > 7 days < 1,200 g 20 mg/kg/day 2 times daily; > 7 days > 1,200 g 30 mg/kg/day 3–4 times daily. Children: Orally 30–50 mg/kg/day in 3–4 divided doses max 250 mg 4 times daily may be given. 12–18 yr: 250–500 mg 4 times daily. IV: 1 month to 18 yr 12.5 mg/kg/dose 4 times daily or as a continuous infusion. Maximum dose: 4 g/day. Replace by oral dosage as soon as possible. Special indications: Topical (acne vulgaris), wash and apply twice daily directly to the affected area. Secondary prevention of rheumatic fever, when child is sensitive to penicillin, oral 20 mg/kg/day max 500 mg twice daily (contraindicated in liver disorder). *Chlamydia trachomatis* pneumonia in infants and neonates: Oral 50 mg/kg/day (erythromycin base) in four divided doses for 14 days. Ophthalmia neonatorum caused by *C. trachomatis*: Neonates, oral 50 mg/kg/day in four divided doses for 14 days. If chlamydial conjunctivitis recurs after discontinuing therapy, the erythromycin dosage regimen should be repeated. A beta-hemolytic streptococcal (GAS) pharyngitis (primary rheumatic fever prophylaxis as an alternative to penicillin in children allergic to penicillin), 40 mg/kg/day in 4 divided doses × 10 days. Cardiology sub chapter of IAP does not recommend using erythromycin for this indication. Uncomplicated urethral, endocervical, or rectal gonorrhea, penicillinase-producing *Neisseria gonorrhoeae*, or for gonorrhea during pregnancy: Adolescent 500 mg PO four times per day for 7 days. Treatment and postexposure pertussis prophylaxis (for postexposure prophylaxis, administer to close contacts within 3 weeks of exposure, especially in high-risk patients (e.g. women in 3rd trimester, infants < 12 months). Oral dosage: Infants, children, and adolescents 40–50 mg/kg/day PO (maximum 2 g/day) in four divided doses for 14 days. For neonates: Azithromycin is the preferred. If azithromycin is unavailable, erythromycin 40–50 mg/kg/day PO in 4 divided doses may be used. Monitor for infantile hypertrophic pyloric stenosis. Pneumococcal prophylaxis: 1 month to 2 yr 250 mg/day, 2–8 yr 500 mg/day, >9 yr 1 g/day in 2 divided doses. Gastric stasis: Oral/IV, 1 month to 18 yr, 3 mg/kg 4 times daily.

Contd...

Contd...

Name	***Formulations***	***Dosage and interval***
Roxithromycin	Tab/DT: 50, 75 150, 300 mg Syr: 50, 100 mg/5 mL	3–4 mg/kg bd
Clarithromycin	Tab: 125, 250, 500 mg Syr: 125 mg/5 mL	Oral 15 mg/kg/24 hrs in 2 divided doses up to maximum of 500 mg twice daily for 5–10 days. *H. pylori* 1–2 yr 125 mg, 2–6 yr 250 mg, 6–9 yr 375 mg, 9–12 yr 500 mg and 12–18 yr 1 g/day in 2 divided doses along with amoxycillin and omeprazole or amoxicillin and lansoprazole or metronidazole and omeprazole. CAP and pharyngitis in children due to *C. pneumoniae*, *Mycoplasma pneumoniae*, or *Streptococcus pneumoniae* give for 10 days. Bacterial endocarditis prophylaxis: 15 mg/kg (single dose max 500 mg) 30–60 minutes before procedure in children and adolescents allergic to penicillin. Treatment and postexposure pertussis prophylaxis: For postexposure prophylaxis, administer to close contacts within 3 weeks of exposure, especially in high-risk patients (e.g. women in 3rd trimester, infants < 12 months). Oral dosage: Infants > 6 months and children: 15 mg/kg/day up to maximum of 500 mg twice daily for 7 days. Not used in neonates. Patients with renal impairment: CrCl > 60 mL/minute: no dosage adjustment needed. CrCl 30– 60 mL/minute: no dosage adjustment needed except in patients receiving concurrent ritonavir. In these patients, reduce the recommended clarithromycin dose by 50%. CrCl < 30 mL/minute: reduce recommended dose by 50%. In patients receiving ritonavir, decrease the recommended clarithromycin dose by 75%.

Contd...

Contd...

Name	***Formulations***	***Dosage and interval***
Azithromycin	Inj: Vials: 30 mL (20 mg/mL) Tab: 1,000, 500, 250, 100 mg Syr: 200, 100 mg/5 mL	Used in chancroid, legionella infections, atypical pneumonia, pertussis, diphtheria as a second choice to penicillins, multidrug-resistant enteric fever 6 months to 12 yrs 10 mg/kg/day once daily for 3 days up to maximum of 200 mg (3–7 yrs), 300 mg (8–11 yrs, 400 mg (12–14 yrs) and 500 mg > 14 yrs. Alternatively, 10 mg/kg/day once on first day followed by 5 mg/kg/day once daily from day 2 to day 5. Group A beta-hemolytic streptococcal (GAS) pharyngitis and tonsillitis (primary prophylaxis of rheumatic fever): 12.5 mg/kg/day single dose for 5 days (not recommended for secondary prophylaxis of rheumatic fever). Chlamydial infection such as nongonococcal urethritis (NGU) or cervicitis due to susceptible strains of chlamydia trachomatis: Adolescents: single dose of 1 g orally. Bacterial endocarditis prophylaxis: 15 mg/kg (single dose max 500 mg) 30–60 minutes before procedure in children and adolescents allergic to penicillin. Treatment and postexposure pertussis prophylaxis (for postexposure prophylaxis, administer to close contacts within 3 weeks of exposure, especially in high-risk patients (e.g. women in 3rd trimester, infants < 12 months). Oral dosage: Infants > 6 months and children: 10 mg/kg/day (maximum 500 mg) on day 1, then 5 mg/kg/day (maximum 250 mg) on days 2–5. Infants < 6 months: 10 mg/kg/day for 5 days. Monitor for infantile hypertrophic pyloric stenosis in infants < 1 month old. Uncomplicated typhoid fever: Orally: Adolescent: 8–10 mg/kg/day once daily for 7 days 1,000 mg on first day, followed by 500 mg once daily for 6 days. Children: 10 mg/kg/day once daily for 7 days or 5-day regimen of 20 mg/kg/day. Continued treatment may be needed to prevent relapse in cryptosporidiosis. STD caused by chlamydia trachomatis: 12–18 yrs 1 g as single dose. Diphtheria: Dose is same but to be given for 14 days. Pertussis: Infants aged <6 months: 10 mg/kg per day for 5 days. Infants and children aged > 6 months: 10 mg/kg (maximum: 500 mg) on day 1, followed by 5 mg/kg per day (maximum: 250 mg) on days 2–5. Multidrug-resistant enteric fever: 10–20 mg/kg/day for 14 days.

Contd...

Contd...

Name	***Formulations***	***Dosage and interval***
Spiramycin	Tab: 1.5 million units (MU) Syr: 0.375 MU/5 mL	Pregnant women with suspected or confirmed toxoplasma infection: 1.5 g (4.5 million international units) orally twice daily until term if the fetus is not infected.
Lincosamides Lincomycin	Inj: 300 mg/mL Cap: 250, 500 mg. Inj: 300, 600. Syr: 125 mg/5 mL	Inj 10 mg/kg od or bd. Oral: 10–20 mg/kg bd
Clindamycin	Cap: 150, 300 mg Inj: 150 mg/mL; Gel/Oint: 1%	Neonates: < 7 days < 2,000 g 10 mg/kg/day divided 12th hrly IV/IM; <7 days > 2,000 g 15 mg/kg/day divided 8th hrly IV/IM; >7 days < 1,200 g 10 mg/kg/day divided 12th hrly IV/IM; 1,200–2,000 g 15 mg/kg/day divided 8th hrly, > 2,000 g 20 mg/kg/day divided 8th hrly IV/IM. Children 10–40 mg/kg/day divided 8th hrly IV/IM or orally. 12–18 yr 150–300 mg up to max of 450 mg/dose 4 times daily. Falciparum malaria (alternate therapy) with 20 mg/kg/day for 5 days. Acne topical application as thin film 2 times daily with lotion and once with gel. Dose adjusted in hepatic failure: Dose reduced and liver function monitored. Not readily removed by dialysis or peritoneal dialysis.
Chloramphenicol	Inj: Vial 1,000 mg Tab/Cap: 250, 500 mg. Syr: 125 mg/5 mL Lotion: 100 mg/mL Eye drops 0.5%, 1% Ear drp 1%, 5%	Neonates < 14 days 12.5 mg/kg/dose twice daily; > 14 days 12.5 mg/kg/dose 2–4 times daily - monitor levels. Children 50 mg/kg/day (maximum 1 g/day) 4 divided doses (double dose for meningitis, septicemia). Ear drops: 2–3 drops 2–3 times daily. Eye ointment may be used in the ear. Eye drops: 1 drop 4–6 times daily (1–2 hrly in severe infections). In addition, a small amount of ointment may be applied at bedtime. Eye ointment: Apply 4 times daily (1–2 hrly in severe infections). Continue treatment till 48 hrs after the eye is clinically normal.

Contd...

Contd...

Name	***Formulations***	***Dosage and interval***
Oxazolidinones Linezolid	Tab: 600, Inj: 2 mg/mL 100 mL and 300 mL	IV infusion over 30–120 minutes. Preterm neonates < 7 days old (gestational age < 34 weeks): 10 mg/kg 12th hrly for 14–28 days, 10 mg/kg 8th hrly in those with a suboptimal clinical response; neonates, infants, and children < 12 yrs: 10 mg/kg 8th hrly for 14–28 days. Linezolid is not recommended for empiric treatment of acute CNS infections. Children exhibit variability in drug clearance and systemic exposure. Those with VP shunts achieve variable CSF therapeutic concentrations; ≥ 12 yrs: 600 mg 12th hrly for 14–28 days. May give aztreonam or aminoglycosides concurrently if indicated. Oral: Adolescents and children ≥ 12 yrs: 600 mg 12th hrly for 10–14 days term neonates, infants, and children < 12 yrs: 10 mg/kg 8th hrly for 10–14 days. Preterm neonates < 7 days old (gestational age < 34 weeks): 10 mg/kg 12th hrly for 10–14 days, 10 mg/kg 8th hrly in those with a suboptimal clinical response.
Tetracyclines Tetracycline	Cap/Tab 250, 500 mg	Acne: Topical application 2 times daily for max 10–12 weeks, may be repeated after 12 weeks interval. Aphthous ulceration: Local mouth wash with contents of 250 mg cap of tetracycline in water 3–4 times daily for 2–3 minutes each time (do not swallow) for 3 days.
Oxytetracycline	Inj: 50 mg/mL Cap: 250, 500 mg Eye Oint: 10 mg/g	Acne: Oral 12–18 yr 250–500 mg/dose 12th hrly. Infections: 250–500 mg/dose 6th hrly.
Demeclocycline	Tab/Cap 150, 300 mg	Age > 8 yr: 3–6 mg/kg bd M = 450

Contd...

Contd...

Name	***Formulations***	***Dosage and interval***
Doxycycline	Cap/Tab/DT 50, 100, 200 Syr: 5 mg/mL, 10 mg/mL	Amebiasis, actinomycosis, brucellosis: > 8 yr age, IV: 45 kg or less: initial dose: 4.4 mg/kg IV on the first day, given in 1 or 2 infusions; maintenance dose: 2.2 to 4.4 mg/kg IV per day, given in 1 or 2 infusions, depending on the severity of the infection more than 45 kg: initial dose: 200 mg IV on the first day, given in 1 or 2 infusions, maintenance dose: 100–200 mg IV per day, depending on the severity of the infection; 200 mg may be given in 1 or 2 infusions, oral: 45 kg or less: initial dose: 4.4 mg/kg orally on the first day, given in 2 divided doses, maintenance dose: 2.2 mg/kg orally per day, given once a day or in 2 divided doses; more severe infections: up to 4.4 mg/kg orally per day. More than 45 kg: initial dose: 200 mg orally on the first day, given in 2 or 4 divided doses; maintenance dose: 100 mg orally per day, given once a day or in 2 divided doses; more severe infections: 100 mg orally every 12 hrs. Acne: initial dose: 100 mg orally twice a day for 3–6 weeks or until improvement occurs, maintenance dose: 50–150 mg orally once a day. Cholera: single dose of 4 mg/kg (max 200 mg), multidrug-resistant *P. falciparum* (resistant to both chloroquine and sulfadoxine-pyrimethamine) with quinine at 3.5 mg/kg once a day for 7 days. Malaria prophylaxis: Short-term chemoprophylaxis (less than 6 weeks): 100 mg daily in adults and 1.5 mg/kg body weight for children more than 8 yrs old. The drug should be started 2 days before travel and continued for 4 weeks after leaving the malarious area. Uncomplicated urethral, endocervical, or rectal infections due to *C. trachomatis*: 100 mg orally twice a day for 7 days.

Contd...

Contd...

Name	***Formulations***	***Dosage and interval***
		Uncomplicated gonorrhea: 100 mg orally twice a day for 7 days. Periodontitis: 20 mg orally twice a day for up to 9 months. Plague: 8 yrs or older: Less than 45 kg: 2.2 mg/kg IV twice a day (maximum 200 mg/day); 45 kg or more: 100 mg IV twice a day. Duration of therapy: 10 days (or until 2 days after fever subsides). Mycoplasma pneumonia: 100 mg orally or IV every 12 hrs for 10 to 21 days. Rocky mountain spotted fever, relapsing fever, or typhus: 100 mg orally or IV twice a day for 7 days. Trachoma: 100 mg orally twice a day for 7 days. Tularemia: 100 mg orally or IV twice a day for 14–21 days. Anthrax postexposure prophylaxis: Less than 45 kg: 2.2 mg/kg orally or IV twice a day; 45 kg or more: 100 mg orally or IV twice a day. Total duration of therapy: 60 days after exposure. Uncomplicated urethral, endocervical, or rectal infections due to *C. trachomatis*, 8 yrs or older: 100 mg orally twice a day for 7 days.
Minocycline	Tab: 100 mg	Oral: 50 mg/dose 2 times daily for minimum of 6 weeks. Paucibacillary leprosy: 50 mg single dose, given as a combination with rifampicin and ofloxacin.
Tigecycline	Inj: 50 mg	1.5 mg/kg loading and then 1 mg/kg bd M = 100 mg
Carbapenems Imipenem-cilastatin	Inj: 500 mg	Newborn: IV 20 mg/kg/dose in the frequency < 7 days, 7–21 days and >21 days at 2 times, 3 times and 4 times daily respectively. Children: IV < 3 months 80 mg/kg/day, 3 months to 12 yr 60 mg/kg/day, 12–18 yr 2 g/day in 4 divided doses (max/dose <12 yr 500 >12 yr 1 g). Children: IV < 3 months 80 mg/kg/day, 3 month to 12 yr 60 mg/kg/day, 12–18 yr 2 g/day in 4 divided doses (max dose < 12 yr 500 > 12 yr 1 g).

Contd...

Contd...

Name	Formulations	Dosage and interval
Meropenem ,	Inj: 500 mg	Newborn: 40 mg/kg/day in 2 divided doses < 7 days and in 3 divided doses > 7 days. Double dose in meningitis and severe infection. Children UTI, gynecological, skin and soft tissue infection: 30 mg/kg in 3 divided doses (max 500 mg/dose). Pneumonia, peritonitis, neutropenia, septicemia: 60 mg/kg/day in 3 divided doses (max 1 g/dose). Meningitis and life-threatening infections: 120 mg/kg/day in 3 divided doses (max 2 g/dose). In renal impairment: CrCl (mL/minute/1.73 m^2) 25–50, give full dose but at 12 hrs intervals, 10–25, 50% dose at 12 hrs intervals < 10–50% dose at 24 hrs interval.
Ertapenem	Inj: 1 g	15 mg/kg bd M = 1,000
Miscellaneous Colistimethate	 Inj: 1 million units/80 mg of salt	 2.6 mg = 1 mg colistin base = 30,000u. IM, IV over 5 minutes: 40,000u/kg (adult 2 million units) 8H, or 1.25–2.5 mg/of colistin base 12H. Nebulized along with oral ciprofloxacin for pseudomonas lung infection in cystic fibrosis: < 1 yr 500,000 units, 1–10 yr 1 million units, >10 yr 2 million units 2 times daily. IV for early pseudomonas infections not cleared by ciprofloxacin and nebulized colistin or moderate-severe infection or multi-resistant strains along with aminoglycoside where other regimens fail.
Polymyxin B	Vial 500,000 U/50 mg (1 mg = 10,000 units)	7,500–12,500 units/kg bd

Contd...

Contd...

Name	***Formulations***	***Dosage and interval***
Furazolidone	Tab: 100 mg Syr: 35 mg/5 mL	Oral 1 month to 12 yr 6 mg/kg/day in 4 divided doses and 12–18 yr 400 mg/day in 4 divided doses. 7–10 days for giardiasis and for 4–6 days after defervescence in typhoid fever.
Nitrofurantoin	Tab: 50, 100 mg	Contraindicated in infants < 3 month age. UTI treatment: 3 month to 12 yr 5–7 mg/kg/day and in 12–18 yr 200–400 mg/day in 4 divided doses. UTI prophylaxis: 1–2.5 mg/kg/day in at bedtime or in 2 divided doses (max 100 mg/24 hrs).
Nitrofurazone	Oint, cream, powder 2%	Apply as per requirement
Fusidic acid	Oint 2%	Apply bd or tds
Mupirocin	Oint, cream 2%	Topical cream: Apply to affected area 3 times daily for up to 10 days; nasal ointment apply to the inner surface of each nostril 2–3 times a day for 5–7 days; ointment-apply to affected area 2–3 times daily for up to 10 days.

(AOM: acute otitis media; bd: twice a day; Cap: capsule; CNS: central nervous system; CrCl: creatinine clearance; CSF: cerebrospinal fluid; CSOM: chronic suppurative otitis media; Drp: drops; DT: dispersible tablet; IM: intramuscular; Inj: injection; IV: intravenous; MRSA: methicillin-resistant *Staphylococcus aureus*; Oint: ointment; PDA: patent ductus arteriosus; STD: sexually transmitted disease; Syr: syrup; Tab: tablet; TB: tuberculosis; tds: thrice in a day; TMP: trimethoprim)

Table 2: Antimycobacterial agents.

Name	*Formulations*	*Dosage and route*
Isoniazid (INH)	Tab: 100, 300	Treatment and prophylaxis of TB 10 mg/kg per day (maximum 300 mg/day). Intermittent regimen: 15 mg/kg (range 12–17 mg/kg). INH prophylaxis in doses of 10 mg/kg/day for 6 months: (a) All asymptomatic contacts (under 6 yrs of age) of a smear positive case, after ruling out active disease and irrespective of their BCG, TST or nutritional status. (b) All HIV infected children who either had a known exposure to an infectious TB case or are tuberculin skin test (TST) positive (≥5 mm induration) but have no active TB disease. (c) All TST positive children who are receiving immunosuppressive therapy (e.g. children with nephrotic syndrome, acute leukemia, etc.). (d) A child born to mother who was diagnosed to have TB in pregnancy should receive prophylaxis for 6 months, provided congenital TB has been ruled out. BCG vaccination can be given at birth even if INH chemoprophylaxis is planned.
Ethambutol (EMB)	Tab: 200, 400,600,800	Dose: 20–25 mg/kg/day (maximum 1,500 mg/day). Tuberculosis: Daily regimen: 20 mg/kg as single morning dose (range 15–25 mg/kg; max dose 1,500 mg/day); intermittent regimen: 30 mg/kg (range 25–30 mg/kg).
Pyrazinamide (PZA)	Tab: 250, 300, 500, 750, 1,000 Suspension 250	Oral children 30–35 mg/kg per 24 hrs as single dose or in two divided doses (max 2 g/day) for the first 2 months of the standard 6 months regimen. 12–18 yrs less than 50 kg 1.5 g/day and more than 50 kg 2 g/day as single dose or in two divided doses (max 2 g/day) for the first 2 months of the standard 6 month regimen. Intermittent regimen: 35 mg/kg/day (range 30–40 mg/kg/day).
Cycloserine	Tab/Cap: 250	Tuberculosis: Oral 10–20 mg/kg/day in 2 divided doses. Max 1 g/day. Adolescent: 250–500 mg twice daily for 2 weeks and then increased to 500 mg to 1 g in divided doses.
Ethionamide	Tab: 250	Dose: 20–25 mg/kg/day (maximum 1,500 mg/day) Tuberculosis: Daily regimen 20 mg/kg as single morning dose (range 15–25 mg/kg; max dose 1,500 mg/day); Intermittent regimen: 30 mg/kg (range 25–30 mg/kg).

Contd...

Contd...

Name	***Formulations***	***Dosage and route***
Para-aminosalicylic acid (PAS)	Granules	Oral: 150 mg/kg/day in 2–3 divided doses. Max 12 g/day
Rifampicin (RMP)	Tab: 100, 150, 200, 300, 450, 600 Syr: 100	To be given in empty stomach. Tuberculosis in combination with other drugs: oral 10 mg/kg (max 600 mg/day) as single morning dose. Meningococcal infection prophylaxis and staphylococcal infections: oral < 5 yr 5 mg/kg/dose and > 1 yr 10 mg/kg/dose (max 600 mg/dose) 2 times daily for 2 days for meningococcal infection prophylaxis and for 10–14 days for staphylococcal infections. *H. influenzae* prophylaxis: oral < 3 months 10 mg/kg and > 3 months 20 mg/kg/dose (max 600 mg/dose) once daily for 4 days. Cholestasis: pruritis 5–10 mg/kg (max 600 mg) once daily. Dose adjustment in liver failure. Avoid altogether, or reduce doses for tuberculosis and prophylaxis to 8 mg/kg daily. Prophylaxis of meningococcal and staphylococcal carrier state: Less than 1 month: 5 mg/kg orally or IV every 12 hrs for 2 days 1 month or older: 10 mg/kg (not to exceed 600 mg/dose) orally or IV every 12 hrs for 2 days.
Dapsone	Tab 100 mg	Leprosy: Oral 1–2 mg/kg/day as single dose in combination with rifampicin. Blistering skin conditions: Start at 500 µg/kg/day and increase or decrease as necessary in 12.5 mg increments. Prophylaxis of *Pneumocystis jiroveci* in HIV: > 1 month: 2 mg/kg/day (up to 100 mg) orally once a day.
Clofazimine	Cap: 50, 100 mg	Multibacillary leprosy (in combination with dapsone and rifampicin), by mouth, adolescent, 50 mg once daily and 300 mg once a month; child 10–14 yrs, 50 mg on alternate days and 150 mg once a month; children < 10 yrs: 1 mg/kg PO once daily plus an additional 6 mg/kg PO once per month in combination with dapsone and rifampin; continue treatment for 12 months. Type 2 lepra reaction (erythema nodosum leprosum), by mouth, adolescent, and child 200–300 mg daily in 2 or 3 divided doses for a maximum of 3 months; 4–6 weeks treatment may be required before any effect is seen.

(BCG: bacillus Calmette–Guérin; Cap: capsule; HIV: human immunodeficiency virus; IV: intravenous; Syr: syrup; Tab: tablet; TB: tuberculosis)

Annexure II: Superbugs

Abhay K Shah

Table 1: Gram-positive superbugs.

Drug	*Condition*	*Side effects*	*Dose*	*Remark*
Vancomycin Bactericidal	In all MRSA	IV infusion-related side effects, nephro- and ototoxic	40–60 mg/kg/day 6 hourly	Major work house antimicrobial
Linezolid Bacteriostatic	SSTI, pneumonia, bone and joint infections	Bone marrow suppression	20 mg/kg/day 12 hourly	Potential for resistance
Clindamycin Bacteriostatic	SSTI, pneumonia, endocarditis	Nausea, vomiting	10–13 mg/kg/dose IV every 6–8 hours 40 mg/kg/day with transition to oral therapy (A-II)	Erythromycin-induced resistance Clindamycin-resistance rate is low (e.g. 10%)
Daptomycin	Endovascular bacteremia	Myalgia, muscle cramps	4 mg/kg/day OD × 7 days	No pediatric data
Tigecycline Bacteriostatic-MRSE, VRE, VRSA, DRSP	SSTI, intra-abdominal infections Not to be used below 8 years age Not to be used for UTI and bacteremia	Elevated CPK Teeth staining, photosensitivity	Children aged 8 to <12 years: 1.2 mg/kg of tigecycline every 12 hours intravenously to a maximum dose of 50 mg every 12 hours for 5–14 days. Adolescents aged 12 to <18 years: 50 mg of tigecycline every 12 hours for 5–14 days	
Quinupristin-dalfopristin	Bacterial endocarditis	Pain at infusion site, myalgia, pruritis	7.5 mg/kg/day IV 12 hourly	No pediatric data

(MRSA: methicillin-resistant *Staphylococcus aureus*; CPK: creatine phosphokinase; DRSP: drug-resistant *Streptococcus pneumoniae*; IV: intravenous; MRSE: methicillin-resistant *Staphylococcus epidermidis*; SSTI: skin and soft-tissue infection; UTI: urinary tract infection; VRE: vancomycin-resistant *Enterococcus*; VRS: vancomycin-resistant *Staphylococcus aureus*)

Table 2: Gram-negative superbugs.

Drug	*Clinical situation*	*Side effects*	*Dose*
Colistin and polymyxin B	• UTI • Bacteremias • VAP • Meningitis In UTI colistin preferred over polymyxin	• Nephrotoxicity (20–40% of patients) • Nephrotoxicity rates may be lower with polymyxin B as compared to colistin (50–60%) • Less frequently reported neurotoxicity and neuromuscular blockade	Colistin: 5 mg CBA/kg (loading dose required) Polymyxin B: 20,000–25,000 international units (2–2.5 mg/kg) (loading dose recommended)
Tigecycline	• Most gram-negatives and anaerobes • Not for *Pseudomonas*	As mentioned earlier	As mentioned earlier

(CBA: colistin base activity; UTI: urinary tract infection; VAP: ventilator-associated pneumonia)

Index

Page numbers followed by '*f*' and '*t*' indicate figures and tables respectively.

B

C

D

E

F

G

H

I

J

K

L

M

N

O

P

Q

R

S

T